Dx/Rx:
Breast Cancer

Diana E. Lake, MD

Attending Physician
Memorial Sloan-Kettering Cancer Center
New York, NY

Clinical Associate Professor
Cornell Weill School of Medicine
New York, NY

Series Editor: Manish A. Shah, MD

Division of GI Oncology
Memorial Sloan-Kettering Cancer Center
New York, NY

D0167086

JONES AND BARTLETT PUBLISHERS
Sudbury, Massachusetts
BOSTON   TORONTO   LONDON   SINGAPORE

World Headquarters
Jones and Bartlett Publishers
40 Tall Pine Drive
Sudbury, MA 01776
978-443-5000
info@jbpub.com
www.jbpub.com

Jones and Bartlett Publishers Canada
6339 Ormindale Way
Mississauga, Ontario L5V 1J2
CANADA

Jones and Bartlett Publishers International
Barb House, Barb Mews
London W6 7PA
UK

Jones and Bartlett's books and products are available through most bookstores
and online booksellers. To contact Jones and Bartlett Publishers directly,
call 800-832-0034, fax 978-443-8000, or visit our website at www.jbpub.com.

Substantial discounts on bulk quantities of Jones and Bartlett's publications are
available to corporations, professional associations, and other qualified organizations.
For details and specific discount information, contact the special sales department
at Jones and Bartlett via the above contact information or send an email to
specialsales@jbpub.com.

Copyright © 2006 by Jones and Bartlett Publishers, Inc.

All rights reserved. No part of the material protected by this copyright may be repro-
duced or utilized in any form, electronic or mechanical, including photocopying,
recording, or by any information storage and retrieval system, without written permission from the copyright owner.

Library of Congress Cataloging-in-Publication Data
Lake, Diana E.
  Dx/Rx. Breast cancer / Diana E. Lake.
    p. ; cm.
  Includes bibliographical references and index.
  ISBN-13: 978-0-7637-2681-2 (pbk.)
  ISBN-10: 0-7637-2681-8
  1. Breast—Cancer—Treatment.
  [DNLM: 1. Breast Neoplasms—therapy—Handbooks.   WP 39 L192d 2006]
I. Title: Breast cancer.   II. Title.
  RC280.B8L272   2006
  616.99'449—dc22
                                                                    2006002401

6048

Production Credits
Executive Publisher: Christopher Davis
Associate Editor: Kathy Richardson
Production Director: Amy Rose
Production Editor: Renée Sekerak
Associate Marketing Manager: Laura Kavigian
Manufacturing Buyer: Therese Connell
Cover Design: Anne Spencer
Composition: ATLIS
Printing and Binding: Malloy, Inc.
Cover Printing: Malloy, Inc.

The authors, editor, and publisher have made every effort to provide accurate information. However, they are not responsible for errors, omissions, or for any outcomes
related to the use of the contents of this book and take no responsibility for the use of
the products described. Treatments and side effects described in this book may not be
applicable to all patients; likewise, some patients may require a dose or experience a
side effect that is not described herein. The reader should confer with his or her own
physician regarding specific treatments and side effects. Drugs and medical devices
are discussed that may have limited availability controlled by the Food and Drug
Administration (FDA) for use only in a research study or clinical trial. The drug information presented has been derived from reference sources, recently published data,
and pharmaceutical research data. Research, clinical practice, and government regula-
tions often change the accepted standard in this field. When consideration is being
given to use of any drug in the clinical setting, the healthcare provider or reader is
responsible for determining FDA status of the drug, reading the package insert,
reviewing prescribing information for the most up-to-date recommendations on dose,
precautions, and contraindications, and determining the appropriate usage for the
product. This is especially important in the case of drugs that are new or seldom used.

Printed in the United States of America
10 09 08 07 06   10 9 8 7 6 5 4 3 2 1

Contents

Editor's Preface

Welcome to the Dx/Rx Oncology series. This is a new series of handbooks focusing on the practical management of common malignancies. The current book, *Dx/Rx: Breast Cancer,* provides an excellent and comprehensive overview of the management of breast cancer in the 21st Century. This handbook uniquely summarizes the results of large clinical trials that directly led to changes in practice, and places these changes in context of current standard management. The bulleted format and concise writing style are easy to follow and allow for quick access to vital and practical management issues to aid in the care of your patient. Dr. Lake does an excellent job condensing the enormous field of breast cancer management into a concise, yet comprehensive handbook that is characteristic of this wonderful new series.

Manish A. Shah, MD

Introduction

Breast cancer represents a significant health problem worldwide. In the United States, it is the most frequently diagnosed cancer, accounting for an estimated 216,000 cases in 2004. It is surpassed only by lung cancer in mortality. Even so, more women are surviving. The death rate from breast cancer is reported to decrease by 2.2% per year. Reasons for this decrease include early detection and more effective treatment.

Treatment strategies have become more global, with many clinical trial results reported as combined analysis. Many European trials are multinational and complement US trials. In this fashion, data and new therapeutic approaches can be readily disseminated, at a faster rate.

This handbook is intended to present all aspects of breast cancer, from pathology and diagnosis to surgery and treatment. We have included recent exciting data in the adjuvant, as well as metastatic, setting that involves monoclonal antibody therapy. Genetic aspects of breast cancer, as well as prevention strategies, are also reviewed.

CHAPTER 1

Epidemiology, Risk Factors, and Screening

■ Epidemiology

- Breast cancer is the most frequently diagnosed cancer in US women. In 2004, an estimated 216,000 women were expected to be diagnosed.[1] Among cancer deaths, breast cancer ranks as the second leading cause of death. In general, in female breast cancer:
  - 75% of cases are diagnosed after the age of 50 years.
  - The disease is the second leading cause of death behind lung and bronchus cancer, although more women are now surviving. Therefore, the natural history of breast cancer is more compatible with that of a chronic illness. There is heterogeneity among patients.
  - The death rate since 1990 is decreasing by 2.2% per year.
    - Possible causes of the decline in death rate include:
      - Early detection
      - More effective treatment
  - Racial influences
    - Caucasian women are more likely to develop breast cancer compared with African American women.
    - African American women are more likely to die from breast cancer than other ethnic or racial groups.
    - From ages 36–69 years, African American women have the highest rate of death from breast cancer. This may be more a socioeconomic than a racial issue, as there are data showing similar outcomes with similar treatment (eg, clinical trial entries). Data are also evolving demonstrating that more women of African American ancestry have a baseloid type of breast cancer, which is more aggressive.[2]

- In the senior population (older than 70 years) death rate from breast cancer is greater in white women than in African American women.
- Male breast cancer
  - Rare (< 1% of all breast cancer)
  - Worse prognosis than for women
  - There is often a delay in diagnosis, which leads to more advanced disease at presentation.
  - Median age at diagnosis is 58–62 years.

■ Risk Factors

- Although the majority of breast cancers are sporadic, there are well-documented risk factors, including
  - Genetics
  - Endocrine factors
  - Dietary factors
  - Environmental exposure
- Genetics[3]
  - Family history is a risk factor for developing breast cancer. In families with multiple affected relatives and a pattern of diagnosis occurring at a young age, along with bilaterality of disease, the probability of genetic inheritance increases. The two genes identified so far that account for the majority of hereditary breast cancers are BRCA1 and BRCA2.
    - BRCA1
      - A tumor suppressor gene cloned on chromosome 17 in 1994
      - More than 700 mutations and sequence variations have been described.
      - Mutations demonstrate autosomal dominant inheritance pattern.
      - Usually seen:
        - in 7% of families with breast cancer only
        - in 4% of families with breast cancer and ovarian cancer
        - in families with onset of breast cancer at a young age, but absent family history the mutation rate ranges from 3.3–8%

- BRCA2
  - Located on chromosome 13, with 300 mutations to date
  - Other cancers associated with BRCA2 mutations include pancreatic cancer, adult leukemia, fallopian tube cancer, male breast cancer, and laryngeal cancer.
- Clinical characteristics associated with BRCA1 and BRCA2 mutations:
  - Autosomal dominant inheritance pattern
  - Younger age at diagnosis
  - Bilateral disease
  - Multiple affected family members
  - Association with other cancer, especially ovarian
- Who should be screened
  - Indications based on risk assessment tools such as Gail model, which takes into account family history, prior biopsies, number of pregnancies, age of first delivery, etc.
    - Family history of breast cancer especially if bilateral disease or diagnosis at an young age. Also consider if there is a family history of ovarian or colon cancer.
  - Important to remember that testing will not detect all mutations
- Implications of screening
  - Therapeutic
    - Prophylactic surgery
    - Chemoprevention
    - Surveillance
  - Other mutations that are less common but are established to be associated with increased risk of breast cancer
    - Germline P53 mutations leading to increased incidence of Li-Fraumeni syndrome (multiple carcinomas and sarcomas)
    - Mutation of chromosome 10q23 (Cowden disease-multiple hamartoma syndrome). By age 50, women with this mutation have a 30–50% risk of breast cancer.

- Women with ataxia-telangiectasia-mutated (ATM) gene have an 11% risk of breast cancer by age 50.
- Endocrine factors
  - Initial enthusiasm for hormone replacement therapy (HRT) has diminished with the data showing no cardiovascular benefit.[4]
    - Benefits of hormone therapy:
      - Reduction in osteoporosis
      - Lowering of cholesterol
    - Risks of HRT[5]:
      - Possible increased risk of breast cancer
        - 10% higher breast cancer risk for each 5 years of use
      - Greater risk with combined estrogen/progesterone product than with estrogen replacement therapy alone
      - Greater risk with sequencing of estrogen → estrogen/progestin than with combined estrogen/progestin
        - Addition of progestin to HRT increases risk compared with therapy with estrogen alone
        - Data are evolving demonstrating safety of HRT in women with hereditary breast cancer syndrome who have undergone prophylactic mastectomy and oophorectomy before age 40, and not later than age 50.[6]
  - Pregnancy
    - Early on transiently increases the probability of breast cancer diagnosis after giving birth
    - Later risk reduction
    - Increased mortality from breast cancer with pregnancy during the first 5 years after diagnosis[7]
  - Other endocrine factors
    - Age at first birth
      - First full-term birth after age 30 increased risk range 2.3-fold.
    - Parity
      - Nulliparous women have a relative risk of breast cancer of 1.4 vs. parous women.
    - Oral contraceptive (OC) use[8]

- Risk with OC use is controversial.
- Epidemiological studies on OC use and breast cancer showed a slight increase in relative probability of a breast cancer diagnosis with current use.
- Increased probability of breast cancer diagnosis OC use before first pregnancy

- Dietary factors
  - Studies have shown no convincing evidence of a relationship between dietary fat intake and breast cancer. Results of the recently evaluated phase III Women's Intervention Nutrition Study (WINS) suggest that lowering dietary fat intake may be associated with improved outcome for postmenopausal women with early-stage breast cancer.[9]
  - A recent report evaluating the effect of statins on the risk of breast cancer in the US female veterans noted a 51% risk reduction, controlling for age, smoking, alcohol use, and diabetes.[10]
  - Alcohol consumption and breast cancer
    - 1.4 relative risk (RR) for each 24 grams of alcohol consumed[11]
- Environmental exposure
  - Radiation is the major environmental risk factor
    - Greatest risk if exposure is before age 40
    - Long latency period
    - The initial association between radiation exposure and breast cancer risk was described in young women who received mantle port radiation as treatment for Hodgkin's disease. There is also a link among the ATM gene, radiation exposure, and breast cancer risk.
  - There are no confirmatory data for a relationship between breast risk and:
    - Pesticide exposure
    - Electromagnetic field exposure
- Clinical relevance of risk factors–facts to include in a detailed history:
  - Prior breast biopsies for benign (ductal carcinoma in situ [DCIS]/atypical ductal hyperplasia [ADH]) and malignant changes

- Family history of breast cancer
  - If a first-degree relative has a history of breast cancer, there is an approximate doubling of the risk of breast cancer. If the family members are a mother and her sister, there is an even higher risk. If there is a history of bilateral breast cancer and/or diagnosis at a young age, the suspicion of a familial aspect to the breast cancer should be raised.
    - Include family information from paternal and maternal side.
  - Ask specifically about breast, ovarian, and gastrointestinal malignancies.
    - Families with a history of breast cancer, especially bilateral disease, male breast cancer, ovarian malignancies and colon cancer, are more apt to be carriers of BRCA1 and BRCA2 gene mutations. Women with germline mutations in one or two of these autosomal dominant genes have a lifetime breast cancer risk of 60–80%.[12]
    - Less than 10% of all breast cancers, however, are caused by BRCA1 and BRCA2 mutations.
- Personal history of breast cancer
- Age at time of first birth
  - Three decades ago, MacMahon and colleagues[13] documented that women having a first birth after age 30 had a breast cancer risk twice as high as women delivering before age 18.
  - In nulliparous women, the risk is similar to that of women delivering after age 30.
  - Questions still remain regarding breast cancer risk and exposure to ovulation-stimulating drugs.
  - Onset of menarche and menopause
    - Those with onset of menarche before age 12 have a risk 50% higher risk than those with onset after age 15.[14]
    - The onset of menopause after age 55 is associated with a relative risk of 2 compared with the risk for women with natural menopause occurring before age 45.[15]

- Bilateral oophorectomy exerts a protective effect, as demonstrated by a 50% reduction in risk in patients having oophorectomy at age 40 or younger in comparison with patients having natural menopause at age 50. This is presumably attributed to the rapid decline in hormone levels following oophorectomy.
- Medication history, especially any use of exogenous hormone replacement therapy or OCs
  - With regard to OCs, a retrospective analysis resulting from pooled data from 54 studies involving 53,297 women with breast cancer and 100,239 without breast cancer found that OC use increased the relative risk by 1.2% with no effect of duration of use,[16] but the risk abated within 10 years of discontinuation.
  - This pooled analysis also demonstrated in patients diagnosed with breast cancer before age 35:
    - Trend of increasing risk with OC use before age 20 (RR of 1.54 before age 20, 1.13 for use beginning after age 20)
    - No consistent data examining the various formulations of oral contraceptives
  - Pooled data concerning HRT use involving 57,705 women with breast cancer and 108,411 without breast cancer worldwide (21 countries)[17] demonstrated:
    - 2.3% increase in risk of breast cancer or a relative risk of 1.5 for use of HRT for 5 or more years (Table 1-1)
  - It is accepted that longer-term use of estrogens for HRT is associated with an increased risk of breast cancer. The question of considerable interest is whether or not the addition of progestins to estrogen alters this risk.
  - In a large overview analysis[18] based on a systematic search of the literature in postmenopausal women (18 observational studies and 8 meta-analyses):
    - Current estrogen use was associated with increased breast cancer risk (RR, .21–1.40).

Table 1-1:   Hormone Replacement Therapy and Incidence of Breast Cancer*[a]

Number of years used	Risk (cases/1,000)
5	2
10	6
15	12

*No excessive risk observed for time frame of 5 or more years after discontinuation.

[a]Collaborative Group on Hormonal Factors in Breast Cancer.

- Risk increased with prolonged duration of use.
- Breast cancer risk increased with the use of estrogen combined with progesterone (Hazard ratio [HR], 1.26).
- The results were confirmed by the Collaborative Group on Hormonal Factors in Breast Cancer.[17] This group also noted that the effect of HRT declined after stopping usage, and by 5–10 years the effect was totally nullified.
- Number of prior pregnancies
- Dietary history
    - Debate persists as to whether diets high in fat are associated with breast cancer risk.
    - A meta-analysis of 12 case-control studies showed a protective effect of high-fiber diets.[19]
- Alcohol consumption[20]
    - Two or more alcoholic drinks per day is associated with an elevated breast cancer risk in a California Teachers Study cohort.
        - Of 103,460 at-risk cohort members, 1,742 were diagnosed with invasive breast cancer.
    - Elevated breast cancer risk most noted with recent consumption of 20 grams or greater of alcohol per day (RR, 1.28).

- Elevation in risk was 32% among post-menopausal women and 21% among peri-menopausal and premenopausal women.
  - Of note, the highest breast cancer risks associated with heavy alcohol consumption were in women on HRT or postmenopausal women with a history of previous breast biopsies for benign disease.
- Prior radiation exposure
  - RR of breast cancer after Hodgkin's disease is reported to be 4.7, with the greatest risk at 18 years posttreatment.
  - Angiosarcomas and sarcomas have been reported in the chest wall irradiated field.
  - There is a linear relationship between dose of radiation and breast cancer risk.
  - There are genetic disorders associated with increased sensitivity to radiation exposure (eg, breast cancer risk in patients carrying the ATM gene, which is associated with an abnormal P53 cellular response to the ionizing radiation-induced DNA damage).

■ Screening

- The rationale for screening is based upon the notion of preventing metastases by early diagnosis and treatment. The current standard screening process consists of:
  - Screening mammogram
  - Self-examination
  - Physician-directed examination (clinical breast exam)
- Mammagraphy
  - The goals of a mammogram are:
    - Early diagnosis in asymptomatic patients
    - Detection of cancer at an early age
  - Two major trials in the 1960s and 80s solidified the role of screening mammographies.
    - The pivotal trial was the Health Insurance Plan (HIP) of New York Screening Project, which took place from 1963–1970. This was a two-arm randomized study involving 62,000 women (Figure 1-1). One half of the study group was screened

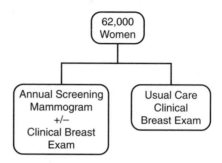

Figure 1-1: Health Insurance Plan of New York Screening Results

➣ 33% of breast cancers were identified by mammography alone
➣ At 10 years, one third reduction in mortality for the screened group in comparison with control
➣ No benefit in screening for women aged 40–49 years*

*A controversial issue for many years. In 2004, the official American Cancer Society guidelines were published.

with mammography and the other half received usual care (defined as clinical breast exam). This was the first trial to demonstrate a screening benefit from mammography alone; one third of the breast cancers detected in this project were found solely with mammography. This trial was also significant for documenting a reduction in mortality at the 10-year period for the 40–49-year-old age group. The study demonstrated a decrease in mortality for women over age 50; this was apparent 5 years following completion of the study.[21]

■ A second major trial, the Breast Cancer Detection Demonstration Project (BCDDP), an NCI- and ACS-sponsored project, was a nonrandomized study involving 283,222 women enrolled between 1973 and 1980. At the commencement of this trial, women younger than age 50 were eligible. However, the early results from the HIP study suggested no benefit for the 40–49-year-old group, and this trial was modified to exclude women younger than

| Age 50–70 | One life would be extended per 1,700–5,000 mammograms |
| Age 40–49 | One life per 5,000–10,000 mammograms would be extended |

Figure 1-2: Benefits of Screening Mammography

age 50 in 1976. However, a 14-year follow-up for the study showed an 80% survival rate in the group of women aged 40–49 years.[21]

- The issue of screening mammography in women younger than age 50 has been debated for several decades. The American Cancer Society has issued the following standardized guidelines on the subject:[22]
  - First screening mammography at age 40, and annually thereafter
  - Clinical breast exam as part of periodic health examination every 3 years for women younger than age 30; annually for women age 40 and older
  - Self-examination starting at age 20
- A meta-analysis of screening studies confirmed that mammography can decrease mortality with annual screening.[23] These results showed that mammography for women aged 40–49 years may be somewhat controversial, but it is beneficial for the 50–60-year-old age group (Figure 1-2).
- Screening for high-risk women
  - BRCA1/BRCA2 mutation abnormalities—start annual mammograms 5 years prior to the age at time of diagnosis of the youngest affected relative

■ References

1.   Jemal A, Tiwari RC, Murray T, et al. Cancer statistics, 2004. *CA Cancer J Clin* 2004;54:8-29.
2.   Study reveals dramatic difference between breast cancers in Caucasian and African women [press release]. Chicago, IL: University of Chicago Medical Center; April 18, 2005.

3. Olapade O, Pichert G. Cancer genetics in oncology practice. *Ann Oncol.* 2001;12:895-908.

4. Waters DD, Alderman EL, Hsia J, et al. Effects of hormone replacement therapy and antioxidant vitamin supplements on coronary atherosclerosis in postmenopausal women: a randomized controlled trial. *JAMA.* 2002;288:2432-2440.

5. Ross RK, Paganini-Hill A, Wan PC, Pike MC. Effect of hormone replacement therapy on breast cancer risk: estrogen versus estrogen plus progestin. *J Natl Cancer Inst.* 2000; 92:328-332.

6. Weber BL. Breast cancer risk assessment: a paradigm for personalized medicine. Plenary session presented at: Annual Meeting of the American Society of Clinical Oncology; May 13-17, 2005; Orlando, FL.

7. Bladstrom A, Anderson H, Olsson H. Worse survival in breast cancer among women with recent childbirth: results from a Swedish population-based register study. *Clin Breast Cancer.* 2003;4:280-285.

8. Romieu I, Berlin JA, Colditz G. Oral contraceptives and breast cancer. Review and meta-analysis. *Cancer.* 1990; 66:2253-2263.

9. Chlebowski RT, Blackburn GL, Elashoff RE, et al. Dietary fat reduction in postmenopausal women with primary breast cancer: phase III Women's Intervention Nutrition Study (WINS). *J Clin Oncol.* 2005;23(suppl):3s.

10. Kochlar R, Khurana V, Bejjanki H, Caldioto G, Fort C. Statins to reduce breast cancer risk: a case control study in U.S. female veterans. *J Clin Oncol.* 2005;23(suppl):7s.

11. Longnecker MP, Berlin JA, Orza MJ, Chalmers TC. A meta-analysis of alcohol consumption in relation to risk of breast cancer. *JAMA.* 1988;260:652-656.

12. Martin AM, Weber BL. Genetic and hormonal risk factors in breast cancer. *J Natl Cancer Inst.* 2000;92:1126-1135.

13. MacMahon B, Cole P, Lin TM, et al. Age at first birth and breast cancer risk. *Bull World Health Organ.* 1970;43:209-221.

14. Titus-Ernstoff L, Longnecker MP, Newcomb PA, et al. Menstrual factors in relation to breast cancer risk. *Cancer Epidemiol Biomarkers Prev.* 1998;7:783-789.

15. Brinton LA, Schairer C, Hoover RN, Fraumeni JF Jr. Menstrual factors and risk of breast cancer. *Cancer Invest.* 1988;6:245-254.

16. Collaborative Group on Hormonal Factors in Breast Cancer. Breast cancer and hormonal contraceptives: collaborative

reanalysis of individual data on 53,297 women with breast cancer and 100,239 women without breast cancer from 54 epidemiological studies. *Lancet.* 1996;347:1713-1727.

17.   Collaborative Group on Hormonal Factors in Breast Cancer. Breast cancer and hormone replacement therapy: collaborative reanalysis of data from 51 epidemiological studies of 52,705 women with breast cancer and 108,411 women without breast cancer. *Lancet.* 1997;350:1047-1059.

18.   Nelson HD, Humphrey LL, Nygren P, Teutsch SM, Allan JD. Postmenopausal hormone replacement therapy: scientific review. *JAMA.* 2002;288:872-881.

19.   Howe GR, Hirohata T, Hislop TG, et al. Dietary factors and risk of breast cancer: combined analysis of 12 case-control studies. *J Natl Cancer Inst.* 1990;82:561-569.

20.   Horn-Ross PL, Canchola AJ, West DW, et al. Patterns of alcohol consumption and breast cancer risk in the California Teachers Study cohort. *Cancer Epidemiol Biomarkers Prev.* 2004;13:405-411.

21.   Dodd GD. American Cancer Society guidelines from the past to the present. *Cancer.* 1993;72(suppl4):1429-1432.

22.   Smith RA, Cokkinides V, Eyre HJ. American Cancer Society guidelines for the early detection of cancer, 2004. *CA Cancer J Clin.* 2004;54:41-52.

23.   National Cancer Institute. Breast cancer (PDQ®): Screening. Available at: wwwcancernetncinihgov 2001. Accessed June 20, 2005.

CHAPTER 2

Diagnostic Tools and Physical Examination

■ Breast Cancer Imaging

- Primary tumor size, and the presence and number of positive axillary nodes are the most important prognostic features in predicting distant metastases from breast cancer. Therefore, early detection is paramount in this regard; multiple imaging techniques are often used to address this goal. These include:
  - Mammography—most sensitive, although 5–10% of cancers detected on mammograms[1] are reported in *Breast Imaging Reporting and Data System (BI-RADS®) Atlas* (Table 2-1)
  - Breast magnetic resonance imaging (MRI)—high sensitivity (94–100%), lower specificity (37–97%)[2]
    - Potential uses of breast MRI (Table 2-2)
      - Standardized technique recently established for breast MRI
    - Interpretation and reporting (see Table 2-1)

■ Physical Examination

- The patient should be carefully examined in the sitting position and with the arms extended overhead while in the supine position. There should be careful examination of the skin; of the lymph nodes in the cervical, supraclavicular, and axillary groups bilaterally, as well as of the breast. Any palpable mass should be measured perpendicularly and its location identified based on a clock position. The mass should be examined for texture (solid vs cystic), fixation, erythema, or edema. Any skin satellite lesions or ulcerations should be described. Nipple/areolar changes should also be described.

Table 2-1: Final Impression MRI and Mammography Categories

BI-RADS category	Interpretation
0	Incomplete, needs additional imaging evaluation
1	Negative
2	Benign finding
3	Probably benign finding, short-term follow-up needed
4	Suspicious, consider biopsy
5	Highly suggestive of malignancy
6	Proven cancer

BI-RADS, Breast Imaging Reporting and Data System.

■ Biopsy Techniques[3,4]

■ Biopsy techniques include fine-needle aspiration, core biopsy, and excisional biopsy (Table 2-3)

■ Additional Diagnostics

■ Indications for bone and/or computed transaxial tomography (CTT) scanning as part of initial staging (Table 2-4)

Table 2-2: Potential Uses of Breast MRI (ASCO 2004)

■ High-risk screening
■ Extent of disease assessment
■ Response to treatment assessment
■ Evaluation of breast implants (Silicone)[a]
■ Identification of an occult primary site in patients presenting with axillary metastases

[a]Morris EA. Review of breast MRI: indications and limitations. *Semin Roentgenol.* 2001:36:226-237.

Table 2-3:   Biopsy Techniques

Type	Advantage	Disadvantage
C Fine-needle aspiration[a]	Rapid, painless, and inexpensive	Cannot distinguish invasive from noninvasive False-negative rate 4–10% False-positive rate <1%
B Core biopsy	Produces histologic details, accuracy similar to fine-needle aspiration Rapid, painless, and inexpensive	False negatives, incomplete characterization of lesions
A Excisional biopsy[b]	Gold standard, complete evaluation of tumor size and histologic characteristics may serve as lumpectomy	Expensive, more painful, may produce cosmetic changes

(A) Must remove a margin of grossly normal tissue around the tumor—1.0 cm or 10 mm is the optimal option. Patients often return for re-excision of positive margins

(B) Radiographics describe probable breast abnormality—core biopsy is procedure of choice

(C) For nonpalpable masses, use ultrasound-guided biopsy

[a]Harris J, Morrow M, Norton L. Malignant tumors of the breast. In: DeVita VT Jr, Hellman S, Rosenberg SA, eds. *Cancer: Principles & Practice of Oncology*. 5th ed. Philadelphia, PA: Lippincott-Raven, 1997:1557-1616.

[b]Silverstein JM, Lagios MD, Groshen S, et al. The influence of margin width on local control of ductal carcinoma in situ of the breast. *N Engl J Med*. 1999;340:1455-1461.

- • Abnormal physical finding
- • Abnormal symptoms
- • Abnormal laboratory function
- ■ Screening tools
  - • Screening with CTT scans of little benefit[3]
  - • Serum tumor markers

Table 2-4:   **Incidence of Metastatic Disease in Patients with Asymptomatic Early-Stage Breast Cancer[a]**

Disease stage	Positive bone scan incidence
I–II	<5%
III	25%

[a]Khansur T, Haick A, Patel B, Balducci L, Vance R, Thigpen T. Evaluation of bone scan as screening work-up in primary and local-regional recurrence of breast cancer. *Am J Clin Oncol.* 1987;10:167-170.

- Carcinoembryonic antigen (CEA)
- CA15-3 (BR27-29)
- Only valuable preoperatively—may be useful in monitoring response
- Valuable preoperatively to assess elevation before the tumor is removed. May also be of value in the metastatic setting—in assessing response to therapy.

■ References

1.   Liberman L. Breast magnetic resonance imaging: technique, interpretation, uses and biopsy. In: *2004 Educational Book.* American Society of Clinical Oncology; 2004:50-56.

2.   Harris J, Morrow M, Norton L. Malignant tumors of the breast. In: DeVita VT Jr, Hellman S, Rosenberg SA, eds. *Cancer: Principles & Practice of Oncology.* 5th ed. Philadelphia, PA: Lippincott-Raven; 1997:1557-1616.

3.   Silverstein MJ, Lagios MD, Groshen S, et al. The influence of margin width on local control of ductal carcinoma in situ of the breast. *N Engl J Med.* 1999;340:1455-1461.

CHAPTER 3

Histopathology, Staging, Natural History, and Pathologic Prognostic Factors

■ Histopathology

- The histological types of breast cancer include:
  - Noninvasive (no penetration of the basement membranes) (Table 3-1)
    - Ductal carcinoma in situ (DCIS)
    - Lobular carcinoma in situ (LCIS—not a true cancer, a marker for risk)
    - Paget's disease
  - Invasive (comprise a heterogenous group, each with a different prognosis)
    - Infiltrating ductal (80%)
    - Infiltrating lobular (10%)
    - Medullary (5%)
    - Mucinous (up to 6%)
    - Tubular (5%)
  - Uncommon
    - Inflammatory
    - Paget's disease
  - Rare
    - Cystosarcoma phyllodes
    - Lymphoma (Table 3-2)
- Nodal status
  - Axillary—nodes most commonly sampled
  - Internal mammary nodes—may be involved in the case of medial lesions
  - Supraclavicular nodes—no longer considered distant metastases
    - Rare site of metastases in absence of axillary or internal mammary nodes

Table 3-1:   Features Distinguishing Noninvasive Lesions

Histology	Mammogram abnormality	Risk
DCIS[a]	Yes (calcifications in mass)	30% risk of invasive disease at 10 years
LCIS[a,b]	No	Marker of risk—37% risk of subsequent invasive carcinoma

[a]Harris J, Morrow M, Norton L. Malignant tumors of the breast. In: DeVita VT Jr, Hellman S, Rosenberg SA, eds. *Cancer: Principles & Practice of Oncology.* 5th ed. Philadelphia, PA: Lippincott-Raven; 1997: 1557-1616.

[b]Henderson I. *American Cancer Society Text Book of Clinical Oncology.* American Cancer Society; 1995.

- Common initial sites of metastases
  - Skin
  - Brain
  - Lung/pleura
  - Bone
  - Liver
    - Common in breast cancer but uncommon as an initial site of metastases

Table 3-2:   1° Lymphoma of the Breast[a,b]

- B-cell lineage
- One half of patients present with large axillary nodes
- Hormone receptors have been described

[a]Mambo NC, Burke JS, Butler JJ. Primary malignant lymphomas of the breast. *Cancer.* 1997;39:2033-2040.

[b]Hugh J, Jackson F, et al. Primary breast lymphoma: an immunohistologic study of 20 new cases. *Cancer.* 1990;66:2602-2611.

- Initial pattern of spread is locoregional, with spread to skin and soft tissue of chest wall, as well as to the axillary and supraclavicular regions.
  - Bone may also be a site of early metastases.
- Metastatic tumors to the breast (Table 3-3)
  - Metastatic tumors to the breast may mimic primary breast cancer, including inflammatory cancer. Most patients, however, already have a known neoplastic history, and metastases to the breast would be compatible with the natural history of the specific cancer.
  - Characteristics of metastatic tumors to the breast
    - Well demarcated
    - Multiple
    - Lack a noninvasive (in situ) component
  - Common metastatic cancers to the breast[1–3]
    - Contralateral breast
    - Lung
    - Malignant melanoma
    - Renal cell
    - Ovarian
    - Gastric
    - Carcinoid

■ Staging

- As of January 2003, the revised American Joint Committee on Cancer (AJCC) staging system for breast cancer was officially adopted for use in tumor registries.[4] A breast task force of international experts was convened to revise the AJCC staging criteria to reflect published clinical data and to be in keeping with current treatment standards. We are becoming more sophisticated with our diagnostic techniques, and more people are partaking in screening, hence we are diagnosing breast cancer lesions earlier and when they are smaller. In spite of this, variable outcomes indicate heterogeneity even within stages. Therefore, changes to the preexisting staging system were evidenced-based and, most importantly, useful for uniform accrual and interpretation of outcome information based on national databases.[4]

Table 3-3:   Tumors Metastatic to the Breast

Study	Number of patients	Tumor reported
Chaignaud[a]	9	3–small cell carcinoma
		2–melanoma
		1–ovarian
		1–carcinoid (lung)
		2–non-Hodgkins lymphomas
Oksufogiv	5	2–rhabdomyosarcoma
		2–ovarian
		1–colon
Nielsen[b]	15	2–thyroid
		2–colon
		3–bronchogenic
		4–melanoma
		1–esophageal
		1–stomach
		1–renal cell
		1–carcinoid
Vergier[c]	8	3–melanoma
		2–rhabdomyosarcoma
		1–mesothelioma
		1–carcinoid
		1–cervical
Domanski[d]	6	1–cervix
		1–endometrial
		1–gastric
		1–small cell lung cancer
		1–large cell lung cancer
		1–myeloma

[a]Chaignaud B, Hall TJ, Powers C, Subramony C, Scott-Conner CE. Diagnosis and natural history of extramammary tumors metastatic to the breast. *J Am Coll Surg.* 1994;179:49-53.

[b]Nielsen M, Andersen JA, Henriksen FW, et al. Metastases to the breast from extramammary carcinomas. *Acta Pathol Microbiol Scand [A]* 1981;89:251-256.

[c]Vergier B, Trojani M, de Mascarel I, Coindre JM, Le Treut A. Metastases to the breast: differential diagnosis from primary breast carcinoma. *J Surg Oncol.* 1991;48:112-116.

[d]Domanski HA. Metastases to the breast from extramammary neoplasms. A report of six cases with diagnosis by fine needle aspiration cytology. *Acta Cytol.* 1996;40:1293-1300.

- The principal changes in the new staging system take into account the widespread use of immunohisto-chemical (IHC) and molecular biologic techniques that afford pathologists the ability to detect micro-scopic lesions down to the isolated tumor cell level (Tables 3-4, 3-5, and 3-6).[4] The changes also reflect the use of sentinel lymph node dissection, which has become the standard of care in the management of early-stage breast cancer. Sentinel lymph node exami-nation incorporates the use of IHC and molecular bio-logic techniques to detect microscopic lesions.

- Despite the new staging system, several questions remain with respect to lymph node metastases (Table 3-7). Pathologists presently agree that the most impor-tant criterion for the potential to metastasize is the size of the lymph node metastasis and not whether it was detected by hematoxylin and eosin (H&E) or IHC staining. Therefore, descriptors are in place in the cur-rent classification system ("i") to describe nodes that are positive by IHC technique but negative by H&E. Likewise, with the advent of molecular biologic tech-niques influencing clinical medicine, reverse tran-scriptase polymerase chain reaction (RT-PCR) can identify single cells. The new staging system, however, designates nodes as pathologically negative if cells are identified by PCR and not by H&E or IHC, but a des-ignator (mol + or −) would be added.

- Five-year survival data[5] in a study of 24,740 patients with breast cancer noted an inverse relationship between the number of positive lymph nodes and overall survival. The revised staging system recognizes the difference in prognosis between patients with 1–3 positive nodes and those with 4 or more. This is now felt to reflect common clinical practice stemming from the 1980 American College of Surgeons (ACS) data documenting a linear decline in survival based on number of positive lymph nodes up to 21.[6] In fact, the early stem cell transplant trials in breast cancer were initiated based on this data.

Table 3-4:   TNM Staging System for Breast Cancer

Primary tumor (T)	
TX	Primary tumor cannot be assessed
T0	No evidence of primary tumor
Tis	Carcinoma in situ
Tis (DCIS)	Ductal carcinoma in situ
Tis (LCIS)	Lobular carcinoma in situ
Tis (Paget)	Paget's disease of the nipple with no tumor Note: Paget's disease associated with a tumor is classified according to the size of the tumor.
T1	Tumor 2 cm in greatest dimension
T1mic	Microinvasion 1 cm in greatest dimension
T1a	Tumor 0.1 cm but not 0.5 cm in greatest dimension
T1b	Tumor 0.5 cm but not 1 cm in greatest dimension
T1c	Tumor 1 cm but not 2 cm in greatest dimension
T2	Tumor 2 cm but not 5 cm in greatest dimension
T3	Tumor 5 cm in greatest dimension
T4	Tumor of any size with direct extension to (a) chest wall or (b) skin, only as described below
T4a	Extension to chest wall, not including pectoralis muscle
T4b	Edema (including peau d'orange) or ulceration of the skin of the breast, or satellite skin nodules confined to the same breast
T4c	Both T4a and T4b
T4d	Inflammatory carcinoma

Table 3-4:   continued

Regional lymph nodes (N)	
NX	Regional lymph nodes cannot be assessed (eg, previously removed)
N0	No regional lymph node metastasis
N1	Metastasis in movable ipsilateral axillary lymph node(s)
N2	Metastases in ipsilateral axillary lymph nodes fixed or matted, or in clinically apparent* ipsilateral internal mammary nodes in the absence of clinically evident axillary lymph node metastasis
N2a	Metastasis in ipsilateral axillary lymph nodes fixed to one another (matted) or to other structures
N2b	Metastasis only in clinically apparent* ipsilateral internal mammary nodes and in the absence of clinically evident axillary lymph node metastasis
N3	Metastasis in ipsilateral infraclavicular lymph node(s), or in clinically apparent* ipsilateral internal mammary lymph node(s) and in the presence of clinically evident axillary lymph node metastasis; or metastasis in ipsilateral supra-clavicular lymph node(s) with or without axillary or internal mammary lymph node involvement
N3a	Metastasis in ipsilateral infraclavicular lymph node(s) and axillary lymph node(s)
N3b	Metastasis in ipsilateral internal mammary lymph node(s) and axillary lymph node(s)
N3c	Metastasis in ipsilateral supraclavicular lymph node(s)

Table 3-4: continued

Regional lymph nodes (pN)[a]	
pNX	Regional lymph nodes cannot be assessed (eg, previously removed or not removed for pathologic study)
pN0	No regional lymph node metastasis histologically, no additional examination for isolated tumor cells Note: Isolated tumor cells (ITC) are defined as single tumor cells or small cell clusters not greater than 0.2 mm, usually detected only by immunohistochemical (IHC) or molecular methods but which may be verified on H&E stains. ITCs do not usually show evidence of malignant activity such as proliferation or stromal reaction.
pN0(i−)	No regional lymph node metastasis histologically, negative IHC
pN0(i+)	No regional lymph node metastasis histologically, positive IHC, no IHC cluster >0.2 mm
pN0(mol−)	No regional lymph node metastasis histologically, negative molecular findings (RT-PCR)[b]
pN0(mol+)	No regional lymph node metastasis histologically, positive molecular findings (RT-PCR)[b]
pN1mi	Micrometastasis (>0.2 mm, none >2.0 mm)
pN1	Metastasis in one to three axillary lymph nodes and/or in internal mammary nodes with microscopic disease detected by sentinel lymph node dissection but not clinically apparent**
pN1a	Metastasis in one to three axillary lymph nodes
pN1b	Metastasis in internal mammary nodes with microscopic disease detected by sentinel lymph node dissection but not clinically apparent

Table 3-4:   continued

Regional lymph nodes (pN)[a]	
pN1c	Metastasis in one to three axillary lymph nodes and in internal mammary lymph nodes with microscopic disease detected by sentinel lymph node dissection but not clinically apparent** (If associated with greater than 3 positive axillary lymph nodes, the internal mammary nodes are classified as pN3b to reflect increase tumor burden)
pN2	Metastasis in four to nine axillary lymph nodes, or in clinically apparent* internal mammary lymph nodes in the absence of axillary lymph node metastasis
pN2a	Metastasis in four to nine axillary lymph nodes (at least one tumor deposit >2.0 mm)
pN2b	Metastasis in clinically apparent* internal mammary lymph nodes in the absence of axillary lymph node metastasis
pN3	Metastasis in 10 or more axillary lymph nodes, or in infraclavicular lymph nodes, or in clinically apparent* ipsilateral internal mammary lymph nodes with clinically negative microscopic metastasis in internal mammary lymph nodes; or in ipsilateral supraclavicular lymph nodes
pN3a	Metastasis in 10 or more axillary lymph nodes (at least one tumor deposit greater than 2.0 mm), or metastases to the infraclavicular lymph nodes
pN3b	Metastasis in clinically apparent* ipsilateral internal mammary lymph nodes in the presence of 1 or more positive axillary lymph nodes; or in more than 3 axillary lymph nodes and in internal mammary lymph nodes with microscopic disease detected by sentinel lymph node dissection but not clinically apparent**

Table 3-4: continued

Regional lymph nodes (pN)[a]	
pN3c	Metastasis in ipsilateral supraclavicular lymph nodes

Used with the permission of the American Joint Committee on Cancer (AJCC), Chicago, Illinois. The original source for this material is the *AJCC Cancer Staging Manual,* Sixth Edition (2002) published by Springer-Verlag, New York, www.springer-ny.com.

*Clinically apparent is defined as detected by imaging studies (excluding lymphoscintigraphy) or by clinical examination or grossly visible pathologically.

[a]Classification is based on axillary lymph node dissection with or without sentinel lymph node dissection. Classification based solely on sentinel lymph node dissection without subsequent axillary lymph node dissection is designated (sn) for "sentinel node," for example, pN0(it)(sn).

[b]RT-PCR: reverse transcriptase/polymerase chain reaction.

**Not clinically apparent is defined as not detected by imaging studies (excluding lymphoscintigraphy) or by clinical examination.

- Location of positive lymph nodes is also of prognostic significance[4,7]
  - Positive infraclavicular lymph nodes (disease-free survival [DFS] rate, 5%; overall survival [OS] rate, 58%)
    - Negative involvement (DFS rate, 68%; OS rate, 83%)
  - Positive supraclavicular lymph nodes (5-year survival rates, 5–34%)[4]
    - With combined-modality treatment, 5-year and 10-year DFS rates were 34% and 32%, respectively,[8] and OS rates were 41% and 31%, respectively. Based on this, metastases to supraclavicular lymph nodes have been reclassified as N3 instead of M1.

Table 3-5: Breast Cancer Stage Grouping

Stage grouping	Primary tumor	Lymph node status	Metastasis
0	Tis	N0	M0
I	T1*	N0	M0
IIA	T0	N1	M0
	T1*	N1	M0
	T2	N0	M0
IIB	T2	N1	M0
	T3	N0	M0
IIIA	T0	N2	M0
	T1*	N2	M0
	T2	N2	M0
	T3	N1	M0
	T3	N2	M0
IIIB	T4	N0	M0
	T4	N1	M0
	T4	N2	M0
IIIC	Any T	N3	M0
IV	Any T	Any N	M1

*T1 includes T1 mic.

Note: Stage designation may be changed if postsurgical imaging studies reveal the presence of distant metastases, provided that the studies are carried out within 4 months of diagnosis in the absence of disease progression and provided that the patient has not received neoadjuvant therapy.

Used with the the permission of the American Joint Committee on Cancer (AJCC), Chicago, Illinois. The original source for this material is the *AJCC Cancer Staging Manual,* Sixth Edition (2002) published by Springer-Verlag, New York, www.springer-ny.com.

Table 3-6: Major Changes in the Staging System

- Discrimination between micrometastases and isolated tumor cells based on size
- Classification of lymph node status by number of positive axillary nodes
- New classification for metastases to the following nodal groups:
  - Infraclavicular
  - Internal mammary
  - Supraclavicular

- A summary of stage grouping for breast cancer can be found in Table 3-4.

■ Prognostic Factors[9] (Table 3-8)

- Tumor size
- Axillary lymph node status
- Histologic grade—may also help identify risk stratification within selective stage
- Histologic subtype (Table 3-9)
- Hormone receptor status
- Human epidermal growth factor receptor 2 (HER-2)/neu overexpression status (Table 3-10)
  - Two most common FDA-approved assay systems for detection of overexpression
    - Fluorescence in situ hybridization (FISH)

Table 3-7: Unanswered Questions Regarding Lymph Node Metastases

- Is there a nodal metastatic size below which lesions are no longer clinically significant?
- What is the clinical significance of IHC-positive-only lymph nodes (IHC positive, H&E negative)?

H&E, hematoxylin and eosin; IHC, immunohistochemical.

Table 3-8: Prognostic Factors

- Tumor size
- Number of positive lymph nodes
- Hormone receptor status
- HER-2/neu (erb B$_2$) overexpression (see Table 3-9)
- Vascular invasion

HER-2, human epidermal growth factor receptor-2.

Table 3-9: Favorable Histologic Subtypes

- Pure tabular
- Pure mucinous
- Medullary

- Expressed as molecules/gene copy ratio ($\geq$2.0 is positive)
  - IHC staining (Dako HercepTest® Kit, DakoCytomation Inc, Carpinteria, CA)
    - Expressed as scoring system (0–3+) in which 3+ correlates best with FISH positivity
  - Best methods are still evolving
- Degree of angiolymphatic invasion
- Other prognostic markers not routinely reported as part of the initial pathology report

Table 3-10: HER-2/neu Overexpressing Tumors

- Found in one third out of all breast cancer cases
- Associated with high histologic grade
- Associated with early metastases
- Suggestion of increased responsiveness to doxorubicin-based regimens
- Possibly less responsiveness to tamoxifen
- May respond better to aromatase inhibitors

- DNA—S-phase analysis
- Mutation of tumor suppressor gene
■ In summary, every pathology report should include the following prognostic features:
  - Tumor size
    ■ Note: Tumor size is usually related to, but is independent of, the lymph node status; tumor size has an effect on prognosis.
  - Lymph node status
  - Histologic grade
    ■ This is based on the amount of nuclear pleomorphism, the degree of tubule formation, and the number of mitoses. Histologic grade usually increases with increasing tumor size and with advancing anatomic stage.
  - Estrogen and progesterone hormone receptor status
  - Presence or absence of vascular/lymphatic invasion (angiolymphatic invasion)
    ■ In multivariate analysis, vascular invasion has been shown to be an independent prognostic factor for both survival and local recurrence.[10]
  - HER-2/neu status
    ■ HER-2/neu is a 185 kDa transmembrane tyrosine kinase. Normally, after HER-2/neu binds to its ligand, the receptor complexes form heterodimers or homodimers. Overexpression of HER-2/neu in breast cancer leads to homodimerization, which leads to activation of the tyrosine kinase region. Activation of kinase-signaling pathways results in changes in cell migration, motility, and survival. Overexpression and amplification of HER-2/neu (one third of breast cancers) correlate with a poor survival and somewhat less response to certain endocrine agents (tamoxifen) and chemotherapy drugs (methotrexate). In 1987, Slamon and colleagues[11] published the pivotal article documenting that HER-2/neu amplification was an independent prognostic factor predicting poor OS or shorter DFS in women with node positive breast cancer.

- Knowledge of HER-2 is important for achieving the following objectives:
  - Establishing prognosis
  - Choosing appropriate hormonal therapy agent (aromatase inhibitor or tamoxifen)
  - Determining eligibility for monoclonal antibody therapy (trastuzumab), which recently has been shown to dramatically improve the time to distant recurrence
    - Demonstrated a 53% reduction in distant metastases at 3 years in a combined analysis of two protocols (National Surgical Adjuvant Breast and Bowel Project [NSABP] B-31 and North Central Cancer Treatment Group [NCCTG]-N983112,13)
- Breast cancer subtypes
  - With the recent development of microarray technology, we are now aware of distinct subtypes of breast cancer arising from different cell types. These subtypes are associated with distinctly different patient outcomes and characteristics. One such subtype, the basal epithelial phenotype, is found in less than 15% of invasive breast cancers.[14] This phenotype is also referred to as "triple negative" or basaloid type breast cancer. It is characterized by the lack of expression of estrogen or progesterone receptors, and the lack of HER-2/neu overexpression. This phenotype is distinctly different from those arising from the inner milk-secreting luminal cells (luminal breast cancer), which accounts for the majority of US and Northern European breast cancer. Researchers have recently begun to describe the basaloid phenotype in association with germline BRCA1 mutations[14] as well as in women of African ancestry.[15] The basaloid phenotype is of independent prognostic value and is an important subtype, as it is associated with a poor prognosis.
  - As we develop more sophisticated technology, our understanding of breast cancer as a heterogenous

group of diseases becomes more clear. Prior to microarray technology, we relied on histologic presentation. With the new technology, we can understand breast cancer as two phenotypes—luminal, more common in US and European women, and basaloid, more common in those with germline BRCA1 mutations and women of African ancestry.

- Therefore, it appears that the estrogen receptor (ER)-negative phenotype can be further subdivided into those with HER-2/neu overexpression and those without (basaloid type).

- Cell type responses to chemotherapy have also been reported, with the basaloid type responding to cytotoxic chemotherapy in a different manner and perhaps being more aggressive.[16]

- Regardless of tumor size and lymph node status, breast cancer derived from the basal epithelial cells of the normal mammary gland is associated with a particularly poor prognosis.

- Large randomized studies have confirmed that the most important prognostic features determining risk are tumor size and lymph node status. A patient with a tumor of 1.0 cm or greater, regardless of the lymph node status, should have a discussion with the medical oncologist regarding the implementation of chemotherapy. In a node-negative patient, a tumor of 1.0 cm can potentially have begun to spread (micrometastases) even though the physical examination and blood chemistries are within normal range. So, chemotherapeutic treatment of patients with no lymph node involvement who have tumors of at least 1 cm can be thought of as treating for presumed micrometastases. Likewise, a patient with a tumor of any size that has spread to a lymph node should be offered chemotherapy, unless there is a contraindication (eg, comorbid conditions, patient refusal). It is also an accepted fact that most patients may benefit from adjuvant chemotherapy. If patients are segregated according to the ER status of their tumors, those with ER-negative tumors will experience a greater degree of benefit than those with ER-positive tumors.

- An especially favorable prognostic group includes patients who have lymph node-negative and hormone-receptor positive breast cancer with small tumors, especially of the favorable histologic types (lobular, mucinous, and papillary). In the current era of gene mapping and molecular profiling technology, this group would be ideal to study to clarify prognosis. This has been done with a 21-gene PCR assay, the Onco-type DX™ (Genomic Health Inc, Redwood City, CA) breast cancer assay.[17]

  - This technology is based on gene expression studies in paraffin-embedded tissue. The investigators surveyed the literature and selected 250 "candidate genes" from published literature databases as well as results from DNA arrays performed on fresh-frozen tissue. From this data, a panel of 16 cancer-related genes and 5 reference genes was selected (Figure 3-1), based on levels of expression of genes. These genes were formulated into an algorithm

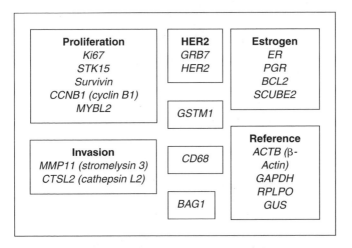

Figure 3-1: Panel of 21 Genes and the Recurrence-Score Algorithm Reprinted from Paik S, Shak S, Tang G, et al. A multigene assay to predict recurrence of Tamoxifen-treated, node-negative breast cancer. *N Engl J Med.* 2004;351:2817–2826. Reprinted with permission Massachusetts Medical Society.

that allows the computation of a recurrence score for each tumor sample. This assay has been validated in the ability to quantify the likelihood of breast cancer recurrence in a significant proportion of early-stage breast cancer and, most importantly, the magnitude of chemotherapy benefit can also be predicted. Therefore, in addition to the standard prognostic features of node status and hormone receptor status, for example, we can now perform a molecular profile on paraffin-embedded tissue from patients with node-negative, ER-positive breast cancer using the assay to obtain a recurrence score that stratifies risk as low, intermediate, or high. The 21-gene panel assay is not only able to quantify breast cancer recurrence risk but is also able to predict response to chemotherapy. The Oncotype DX™ assay has been validated by NSABP studies (B-14, breast cancer recurrence study; B-20, chemotherapy benefit study).

- The objective of the B-14 trial was to validate recurrence score as a predictor of distant recurrence in node-negative, ER-positive breast cancer in tamoxifen-treated patients (Figure 3-2).

- Those randomized to tamoxifen were registered on the Genomic Health/NSABP B-14 prospective clinical validation study.

- The primary end point was distant recurrence-free survival; secondary end points were relapse-free survival and OS.

- The B-14 trial results validated that the distant recurrence-free survival in the low-risk group (recurrence score of less than 18) was signifi-

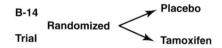

Figure 3-2: NSABP B-14 Trial Design
NSABP, National Surgical Adjuvant Breast and Bowel Project.

cantly lower than the 10-year distant relapse-free survival in the high-risk group (recurrence score of 31 or higher). Ten-year recurrence rate was 6.8% in the low-risk group patients in contrast to 30.5% in the high-risk group ($P<0.00001$).

- It was shown that the recurrence score was better than standard measures of age, tumor size, and tumor grade as a prognostic indicator for the risk of distant recurrence.[17]

■ Although adjuvant chemotherapy has been proven to be beneficial in most patients, in some patients it will result in overtreatment and expose them to unnecessary toxicity. If a patient presents with breast cancer features that invoke a conversation regarding chemotherapy and the patient is hesitant to accept treatment, this type of assay can be beneficial.

■ References

1   Hadju S, Urloun J. Cancers metastatic to the breast. *Cancer*. 1968;22:1691-1696.

2. Nielsen M, Anderson JA, Henriken FW, et al. Metastases to the breast from extramammary carcinomas. *Acta Pathol Microbiol Scand [A]*. 1981;89:251-256.

3. Harris T, Kalisher J. Breast metastases: an unusual manifestation of a malignant carcinoid tumor. *Cancer*. 1977;40:3102-3106.

4. Singletary SE, Allred C, Ashley P, et al. Revision of the American Joint Committee on Cancer staging system for breast cancer. *J Clin Oncol*. 2002;20:3628-3636.

5. Carter C, Allen C, Henson D. Relation of tumor size, lymph node status, and survival in 24,740 breast cancer cases. *Cancer*. 1988;63:181-185.

6. Nemoto T, Vana J, Bedwani RN, Baker HW, McGregor FH, Murphy GP. Management and survival of female breast cancer: results of a national survey by the American College of Surgeons. *Cancer*. 1980;45:2917-2924.

7. Newman LA, Kuerer HM, Fornage B, et al. Adverse prognostic significance of infraclavicular lymph nodes detected by ultrasonography in patients with locally advanced breast cancer. *Am J Surg*. 2001;181:313-318.

8. Brito RA, Valero V, Buzdar AU, et al. Long-term results of combined-modality therapy for locally advanced breast cancer with ipsilateral supraclavicular metastases: The University of Texas M.D. Anderson Cancer Center experience. *J Clin Oncol.* 2001;19:628-633.

9. Fitzgibbons PL, Page DL, Weaver D, et al. Prognostic factors in breast cancer. College of American Pathologists Consensus Statement 1999. *Arch Pathol Lab Med.* 2000;124:966-978.

10. Pinder SE, Ellis IO, Galea M, O'Rouke S, Blamey RW, Elston CW. Pathological prognostic factors in breast cancer. III. Vascular invasion: relationship with recurrence and survival in a large study with long-term follow-up. *Histopathology.* 1994;24:41-47.

11. Slamon DJ, Clark GM, Wong SG, Levin WJ, Ullrich A, McGuire WL. Human breast cancer: correlation of relapse and survival with amplification of the HER-2/neu oncogene. *Science.* 1987;235:177-182.

12. Romond EH, Perez E, Bryant J, Suman V, et al. Doxorubicin & cyclophosphamide followed by paclitaxel with or without trastuzumab as adjuvant therapy for patients with HER2-positive operable breast cancer: combined analysis of NSABP-B31/NCCTG N9831. In press. Paper presented at: Annual Meeting of American Society of Clinical Oncology; May 15, 2005; Orlando, FL.

13. Perez E, Suman V, Davidson N, et al. Interim cardiac safety anaylsis of NCCTG N9831 Intergroup adjuvant trastuzumab trial. *J Clin Oncol.* 2005;23(suppl):17s.

14. Foulkes WD, Stefansson IM, Chappuis PO, et al. Germline BRCA1 mutations and a basal epithelial phenotype in breast cancer. *J Natl Cancer Inst.* 2003;95:1482-1485.

15. Study reveals dramatic difference. Chicago, IL: University of Chicago Medical Center; April 18, 2005.

16. Troester MA, Hoadley KA, Sorlie T, et al. Cell-type-specific responses to chemotherapeutics in breast cancer. *Cancer Res.* 2004;64:4218-4226.

17. Paik S, Shak S, Tang G, et al. A multigene assay to predict recurrence of tamoxifen-treated, node-negative breast cancer. *N Engl J Med.* 2004;351:2817-2826.

CHAPTER 4

Surgical Management of Breast Cancer: Ductal Carcinoma In Situ and Invasive Disease

■ Surgical Management

- Initial evaluation
  - Patients usually present with an abnormal screening radiographic study or a palpable abnormality. It should be noted that any suspicious abnormality warrants investigation to make a diagnosis. Such diagnostic techniques have been discussed earlier. If the biopsy reveals a benign abnormality, appropriate follow-up is required. For malignancy, surgical management depends on whether noninvasive or invasive breast cancer is diagnosed.
- DCIS
  - Surgical options
    - Wide excision with or without radiation therapy
    - Simple mastectomy (Table 4-1)
  - For DCIS lesions detected as calcifications, a postoperative mammogram should be performed to ensure that no calcifications remain.
- DCIS and axillary node dissection
  - Not required if there is no evidence of invasion
  - If there is concern that an invasive component may be found, lymphoscintigraphy may be performed.
  - A small number of cases (6–13%) have micrometastases[1]
- High-risk LCIS and atypical ductal hyperplasia
  - Finding either on biopsy is not an indication for surgery.
  - LCIS at surgical margin does not require excision of margin.

Table 4-1:   Absolute Indications for Total Mastectomy

- Inability to completely excise tumor
- Multicentric disease
- A contraindication to radiation therapy

- Invasive breast cancer
  - Surgical goals
    - Definitive local control
      - Wide excision with sentinel lymph node (SLN) mapping and biopsy with or without axillary lymph node dissection if SLN is positive
      - Mastectomy
      - Wide excision without axillary lymph node dissection in select cases (elderly)
      - Surgical margins must be free of cancer (3–4 mm) (DCIS or invasive disease).
      - Lumpectomy is surgical procedure of choice, unless contraindicated (Table 4-2).
- Prophylactic mastectomy
  - Consider in patients at high risk for developing breast cancer
  - Total mastectomy, including nipple areola complex, is operation of choice
- Subcutaneous mastectomy
  - No role

Table 4-2:   Contraindications to Breast-Conserving Surgery

- Active collagen vascular disease precluding radiation
- Multicentric tumor
- First- or second-trimester pregnancy
- Past history of breast irradiation
- Pacemaker in radiation port that cannot be moved
- Morbid obesity exceeding structural load capacity of radiotherapy table
- Diffuse abnormal microcalcifications in mammogram (malignant appearing or indeterminate)
- Inability to completely excise primary tumor with clear margins

- Breast reconstruction
  - Consider in patients requiring mastectomy
  - Determine suitability based on evaluation by surgical oncologist and plastic reconstructive surgeon, and on patient preference
  - Consider need for postoperative radiation in timing of surgery

■ Reference

1.   Pendas S, Dauway E, Giuliano R, Ku N, Cox CE, Reintgen DS. Sentinel node biopsy in ductal carcinoma in situ patients. *Ann Surg Oncol.* 2000;7:15-20.

CHAPTER 5

Systemic Adjuvant Therapy for Early-Stage Breast Cancer

▪ Systemic or Medical Management

- Assessment of disease progression
  - Following a diagnosis of primary breast cancer, the appropriate assessment includes:
    - Complete blood count
    - Chemistry profile, including liver function tests
    - Chest x-ray
    - Bilateral mammography
    - Bone scan, CTTs, and MRIs
      - In selected clinical settings, based on history, symptoms, physical examination, and/or abnormal chemistries
- Adjuvant systematic therapy
  - A decision concerning the benefit and choice of adjuvant systemic therapy should be made based on the pathologic characteristics of the tumor, including:
    - Tumor size
    - Lymph node status
    - Hormone receptor status
    - Degree of angiolymphatic invasion
    - HER-2/neu overexpression status
  - May also consider basing decision on Oncotype Dx™ score
    - Less than 18—low risk for distant recurrence and, therefore, least benefit from chemotherapy
    - 18–30—intermediate risk
    - 31 or greater—high risk for distant recurrence and greatest benefit from chemotherapy
  - The Early Breast Cancer Trialists' Collaborative Group analysis of adjuvant therapies has demonstrated a clear benefit from adjuvant systemic therapy.

More significant is the fact that the earlier distinction between premenopausal and postmenopausal women is less important and has been superseded by the distinction between estrogen receptor values, regardless of the menopausal status.[1]

- Results of the Early Breast Cancer Trialists' Collaborative Group (EBCTCG) consensus meeting November 2000[2] (updated 2005[3]) concerning adjuvant endocrine therapy
  - Measurement of 10 fmol or greater of estrogen receptor protein per mg cytosol protein was considered ER positive or, if not measured, any IHC evidence of estrogen receptor protein was considered ER positive[3,4]
  - Patients with insufficient tissue should be considered as having ER-positive tumors.
  - Patients with ER-negative/progesterone receptor (PR)-positive tumors may benefit.
  - HER-2/neu overexpression is not a deterrent to using tamoxifen[2] (controversial).

■ Endocrine Drug Therapy (Tables 5-1 and 5-2)

- The goal of endocrine therapy is to block the effect of estrogen at the cellular level. This can be achieved by several mechanisms. Selective estrogen receptor modulators (SERMS) include tamoxifen and raloxifene, and selective estrogen receptor down modulators (SERDs) include fulvestrant. A newer class of drugs, the aromatase inhibitors (eg, anastrozole, letrozole, exemestane), block estrogen production at the tissue level by inhibiting reversibly or irreversibly the aromatase enzyme.
- Premenopausal women may be treated with tamoxifen. Aromatase inhibitors are restricted to postmenopausal patients (Table 5-3).
- Third-generation aromatase inhibitors (letrozole, anastrozole, exemestane)[5]
  - Decrease in serum estrogen levels to 1–10% of pretreatment levels

Table 5-1:   Mechanisms of Action of Endocrine Therapies

- Lower estrogen levels (oophorectomy, aromatase inhibitors)
- Modulate estrogen receptors (SERMS, tamoxifen, toremifene)
- Modulate estrogen receptors with pure agonist activity (ER down-modulator fulvestrant)
- High-dose estrogens, progestins, androgens have activity against ER+ tumors: mechanism of action is unclear.

- Less toxicities than earlier agents (aminogluthemide, megestrol)
- Earlier aromatase inhibitors unable to suppress estrogen levels in premenopausal women
- Combining a third-generation aromatase inhibitor with ovarian suppression using a luteinizing hormone releasing hormone (LHRH) may be effective in premenopausal women.

■ Adjuvant endocrine therapy
- Oxford overview analysis[1]
  ■ Data for over 37,000 patients treated with tamoxifen
  ■ Data from 55 trials reviewed
  ■ Follow up for 10 years or more
  ■ Tamoxifen therapy for 5 years was the gold standard (Table 5-4)

■ Duration of tamoxifen therapy (Tables 5-5, 5-6, and 5-7)
- 5 years optimal—in ER-positive disease, the annual death rate from breast cancer is reduced by 31%[3]
- 2 years suboptimal

Table 5-2:   Third-Generation Aromatase Inhibitors[a]

Steroidal type I	Nonsteroidal type II
Exemestane	Anastrozole
	Letrozole

[a]Lake DE, Hudis C. Aromatase inhibitors in breast cancer: an update. *Cancer Control*. 2002;9:490-498.

Table 5-3: Endocrine Therapy Options in Postmenopausal Women

- Aromatase inhibitors alone[a,b]
- Tamoxifen for 5 years
- Tamoxifen for 5 years followed by letrozole for 5 years[c,d]
- Tamoxifen for 2–3 years followed by anastrozole for up to 5 years[e]
- Tamoxifen for 2–3 years followed by exemestane for up to 5 years in total[f]

[a]Baum M, Budzar AU, Cuzick J, et al. Anastrozole alone or in combination with tamoxifen versus tamoxifen alone for adjuvant treatment of postmenopausal women with early breast cancer: first results of the ATAC randomized trial. *Lancet.* 2002; 359:2131-2139.

[b]Baum M, Budzar AU, Cuzick J, et al. Anastrozole or in combination with tamoxifen versus tamoxifen alone for adjuvant treatment of post-menopausal women with early-stage breast cancer: results of the ATAC (Arimidex, Tamoxifen Alone or in Combination) trial efficacy and safety update analyses. *Cancer.* 2003;98:1802-1810.

[c]Goss PE, Ingle JN, Martino S, et al. A randomized trial of letrozole in postmenopausal women after five years of tamoxifen therapy for early-stage breast cancer. *N Engl J Med.* 2003;349:1793-1802.

[d]Goss PE, Ingle JN, Martino S, Robert NJ, et al. Updated analysis of the NCIC CTG MA1.17 randomized placebo (P) controlled trial of letrozole (L) after five years of tamoxifen in postmenopausal women with early stage breast cancer [abstract]. *Proc Am Soc Clin Oncol.* 2004;23:87. Abstract 847.

[e]Boccardo F, Rubagotti A, Amoroso DI, et al. Anastrozole appears to be superior to tamoxifen in women already receiving adjuvant tamoxifen therapy [abstract]. *Breast Cancer Res Treat.* 2003;82(suppl 1):3. Abstract 3.

[f]Coombes RC, Hall E, Gibson LJ, et al. A randomized trial of exemestane after two to three years of tamoxifen therapy in postmenopausal women with primary breast cancer. *N Engl J Med.* 2004;350:1081-1092.

Table 5-4: Additional Benefits from Tamoxifen

- Lipid lowering
- Prevention of postmenopausal bone loss
- Risk reduction in the incidence of contralateral breast cancer

Table 5-5: **ER+ Cancer: Proportional Risk Reduction with Tamoxifen Therapy**

Treatment duration	Recurrence (%)	Mortality (%)
1 year	21	12
2 years	29	17
5 years	47	26

ER+, estrogen receptor-positive.

- Potential benefit of longer treatment must be determined by weighing the toxicity profile of the drug (see Table 5-6) against the risk of recurrence based on features of the tumor.
- Benefits of tamoxifen (see Table 5-4)
  - Risk reduction in mortality from breast cancer

Table 5-6: **ER+ or ER-Poor Cancers*: Contralateral Breast Cancer Risk Reduction with Tamoxifen Therapy[a]**

Treatment duration	Risk (%)
1 year	13
2 years	26
5 years	47

■ Patients with truly ER-negative disease (less than 50) show no benefit from tamoxifen

■ 5 years of tamoxifen is better than 1–2 years (recurrence rate ratio, 0.82, breast cancer death rate ratio, 0.91)

■ Suggestion that ER-poor but progesterone-positive disease may identify a tamoxifen-responsive subset

[a]Early Breast Cancer Trialists' Collaborative Group. Effects of chemotherapy and hormonal therapy for early breast cancer or recurrence and a 15-year survival: an overview of the randomized trials. *Lancet.* 2005;365:1687-1717.

Table 5-7:   Years of Tamoxifen Duration and Disease-Free Survival (DFS) and Overall Survival (OS)

	Tamoxifen 10 yrs	Tamoxifen 5 yrs
NSABP[a]	69% DFS 80% OS	57% DFS 76% OS
ECOG[b]	86% DFS 94% OS	92% DFS 96% OS
Scottish Cancer Trials*[c]	64% DFS	66% DFS

DFS = 5 yr DFS

*Small sample size, allowed concluding only if continuing tamoxifen beyond 5 years is beneficial. The extent of the benefit is modest and not comparable with the benefits noted in the initial 5 years of therapy.

DFS, disease-free survival; OS, overall survival.

[a]Fisher B, Dignam J, Bryant J, et al. Five versus more than five years of tamoxifen therapy for breast cancer patients with negative lymph nodes and estrogen receptor-positive tumors. *J Nat Cancer Inst.* 1996;88:1529-1542.

[b]Tormey D, Gray R, Falkson H. Postchemotherapy adjuvant tamoxifen beyond five years in patients with lymph node-positive breast cancer. *J Natl Cancer Inst.* 1996;88:1828-1833.

[c]Steward HJ, Forrest AP, Everington D, et al. Randomised comparison of 5 years of adjuvant tamoxifen with continuous therapy for operable breast cancer. The Scottish Cancer Trials Breast Group. *Br J Cancer.* 1996;74:297-299.

- Risk reduction in contralateral breast cancer
  - Toxicities associated with tamoxifen (Table 5-8)
    - 5 years of tamoxifen, in comparison with 1–2 years, is associated with a recurrence rate ratio of 0.82 and a death rate ratio of 0.91[3]
- Endometrial cancer and tamoxifen[6]
  - Risk doubled with 1–2 years of adjuvant tamoxifen, but no excess mortality from endometrial cancer resulted with longer treatment[3]
  - Risk increased by a factor of four with 5 years of therapy (1/1,000 women annually)[7]

Table 5-8:   Toxicities Associated with Tamoxifen Therapy

Common	Less common
Hot flushes	Visual disturbances
Vaginal discharge	Ovarian cysts
Endometrial hyperplasia	Keratopathy
Irregular menses	Optic neuritis
	Retinopathy
	Endometrial cancer
	Cataract formation

- The increase in endometrial cancer risk is outweighed by the positive effect of a reduction in contralateral breast cancer.
- Endometrial hyperplasia is a precursor to endometrial cancer.
- Hyperplasia with cytologic atypia represents the greatest risk.
- Unopposed estrogen from any source is a risk factor for developing hyperplasia.
- Abnormal uterine bleeding is the most common presenting symptom.
- Raloxifene (a SERM) is not associated with increased risk.
- Ultrasound (transvaginal) is a good screening tool.[8]

■ Trials of aromatase inhibitors
  - Arimidex, Tamoxifen, Alone or in Combination (ATAC) trial[9,10] (Figure 5-1)
    ■ Double-blind study of 9,366 postmenopausal patients with the following conclusions about anastrozole (Arimidex):
      - Superior DFS at 3 years (89.4% vs. 87.4%)
      - Favorable toxicity profile (Table 5-9)
      - 60% reduction in risk of new contralateral breast cancer
      - Associated with fewer recurrences
      - Greater differential efficacy between anastrozole and tamoxifen in patients with ER-positive

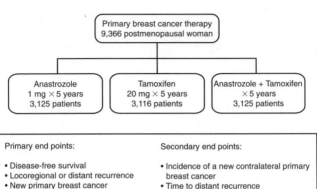

Figure 5-1: ATAC Trial

ATAC, Arimidex, Tamoxifen, Alone or in Combination.

and PR-negative tumors than in those with ER/PR-positive tumors in subset analysis

- MA-17 letrozole trial[11] (Figure 5-2)
  - Event-driven analysis
  - Median follow-up 30 months
  - At 4 years relapse-free survival (RFS) 89.8% with placebo; 94.7% with letrozole
  - Equally effective in node-positive and node-negative disease

Table 5-9: ATAC Trial Tolerability

- All treatments generally well tolerated
- No toxicity data on the combination arm
- Anastrozole significantly better tolerated with respect to:
  - Endometrial cancer
  - Vaginal bleeding
  - Vaginal discharge
  - Ischemic cerebrovascular events
  - Hot flushes
  - Weight gain
- Tamoxifen better tolerated with respect to:
  - Musculoskeletal disorders
  - Fractures

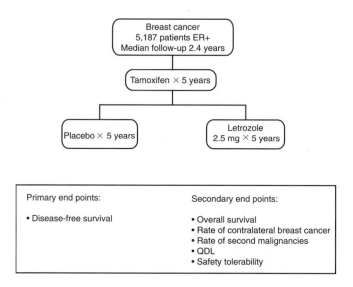

Figure 5-2: MA-17 Letrozole Extended Adjuvant Therapy Trial

- Risk of recurrence reduced by 42%
- Improvement in 3-year DFS regardless of node status (node negative, 3%; node positive, 7%)
- OS benefit demonstrated in node-positive patients (39% decrease in mortality)[11]
- MA-17 trial questions
  - Absolute benefit of letrozole at 5 years is unknown
  - Planned rerandomization to placebo or to 5 additional years of letrozole has begun—will provide data from 15 years of adjuvant endocrine therapy use by patients
- Breast Cancer International Study Group (BIG I)-98
  - Worldwide collaborative effort
  - Four-arm randomized study (Figure 5-3)
  - Findings in primary analysis comparing letrozole with tamoxifen in 8,010 patients
    - Letrozole significantly prolonged 5-year DFS and reduced the risk of recurrence by 15%.
    - Letrozole reduced the risk of distant metastases.

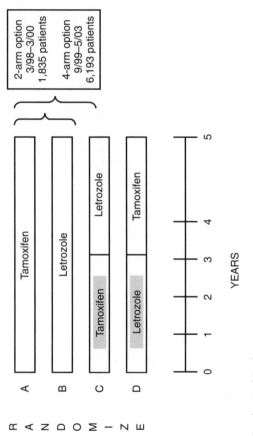

Figure 5-3: Four-Arm Randomized Study

- Letrozole was well tolerated.
- Letrozole reduced the mortality risk by 14%.
- Letrozole demonstrated significant benefit in node-positive patients.
  - Therefore, it seems that no matter when you begin an aromatase inhibitor, following 5 years of tamoxifen, or after 2–3 years of tamoxifen, the results are favorable with the aromatase inhibitor compared with tamoxifen alone.
- Issues with aromatase inhibitors
  - Bone mineral density (BMD)
    - Anastrazole was associated with bone loss in the spine and hip (2-year analysis).[12]
    - Tamoxifen was associated with BMD increase.
    - MA-17 trial—increased incidence of new-onset osteoporosis with letrozole compared with placebo (5.8% vs. 4.5%, respectively)[11]
      - No difference in fracture rate
        - Letrozole, 5.3%
        - Placebo, 4.6%
    - Exemestane (a steroidal aromatase inhibitor) was associated with increased BMD loss in the femoral neck but with no increased risk of fracture or osteoporosis, in comparison with placebo.[13]
  - Lipid levels[14]
    - Tamoxifen—reduces serum cholesterol, may increase triglycerides
    - Anastrazole—no change in total cholesterol or low-density lipids
    - Anastrazole—beneficial change in high-density lipoproteins and in triglycerides
  - Is one aromatase inhibitor more efficacious than another?
    - Presently there is no difference between the two nonsteroidal aromatase inhibitors (anastrazole, letrozole).
      - An open-label, head-to-head, multicenter, multinational, phase III trial coaring letrozole with anastrozole in postmenopausal women with hormone receptor-positive or unknown

metastatic breast cancer failed to show differences in time to progression, OS, or duration of tumor response (Figure 5-4).[15]

- Patient characteristics
  - Hormone receptor-positive (HR-positive) or unknown
  - Metastatic disease
  - Progression on prior antiestrogen therapy
- Primary end point
  - Time to progression (TTP)
- Secondary end points
  - Overall survival (OS)
  - Duration of tumor response (DTR)

	Letrozole	Anastrozole
TTP (mo)	5.7	5.7
Medin OS (mo)	22.0	20.3
DTR (mo)	22	25

Figure 5-4: Letrozole Compared with Anastrozole

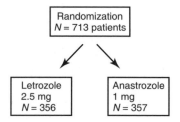

Reprinted from Rose C, Hansen P, Dombernowsky P, et al. A randomized DBCG trial of adjuvent (adj) tamoxifen (TAM) + radiotherapy (RT vs TAM alone vs TAM + CMF in postmenopausal breast cancer patients (pts) with high risk of recurrence [abstract]. *Eur J Cancer.* 1994;30A:S28-S28.

■ Adjuvant Systemic Chemotherapy (Table 5-10)

■ Consider after local surgical management for early-stage breast cancer

Table 5-10:   EBCTCG Adjuvant Polychemotherapy Benefits Summary*

- Reduces contralateral breast cancer by 20%
- No advantage with greater than 6 months polychemotherapy
- Anthracycline-based regimens associated with slightly better 5-year survival rate (72% vs. 69%)
- 3–6 months polychemotherapy yields an absolute improvement in survival rates (7–11% in women <50 years of age; 2–3% in women 50–69 years of age)

EBCTCG, Early Breast Cancer Trialists' Collaborative Group.

*Early Breast Cancer Trialists' Collaborative Group. Polychemotherapy for early breast cancer: an overview of the randomized trials. *Lancet.* 1998;352:930-942.

- Early Breast Cancer Trialists' Collaborative Group analysis of polychemotherapy demonstrated a reduction in odds of recurrence and death.[16]
  - Reduction in recurrence
    - 35% in women younger than age 50–69
    - 20% in women aged 50–69 years
  - Reduction in risk of death
    - 27% in women younger than age 50
    - 11% in women aged 50–69 years
  - Recurrence reduction was mainly in the first 5 years.
  - Survival benefit was within first 10 years.
  - Similar results in node-negative and node-positive patients
  - Absolute mortality benefit of 7% in node-negative patients and 11% in node-positive patients[16]
  - Chemotherapy benefits were independent of menopausal status, age, or prior treatment.
- Factors to consider in the adjuvant chemotherapy treatment decision
  - Reduction in risk of recurrence and survival
  - Toxicities
  - Quality of life
  - Comorbid conditions, especially in the older-than-50 age group

- Candidates for adjuvant chemotherapy include:
  - Patients with lymph node involvement
  - Patients with tumors greater than or equal to 1 cm in greatest diameter, with either lobular or ductal histology
  - Patients with node-negative, hormone receptor-negative tumors or tumors judged to be at high risk for recurrence
  - Little data exist on adjuvant chemotherapy in the older-than-70 age group, however, age alone should not influence decision to administer polychemotherapy.
- Role of anthracyclines
  - Minimum standard of care in node-positive disease
  - 1998 International Consensus Panel on the Treatment of Primary Breast Cancer in St. Gallen, Switzerland,[17] agreed that anthracycline-based regimens were superior to cyclophosphamide, methotrexate, and 5-fluorouracil (CMF).
  - Oxford overview[18] and EBCTCG update[3]—3% absolute survival and recurrence benefit with anthracycline-based regimens compared with CMF at 5 years, and 4% benefit at 10 years
- Role of taxanes (Figure 5-5)
  - Considered among the drugs most active against breast cancer in the metastatic setting
  - Three large randomized trials
    - The pivotal Cancer and Leukemia Group B (CALGB) protocol 9344[19] was a randomization of three dose schedules of doxorubicin (A) (60 mg, 75 mg, and 90 mg), along with cyclophosphamide (C) standard dose (600 mg/m^2) for four cycles at 3-week intervals. At the completion of AC, patients were then randomized to receive paclitaxel for four cycles or to receive no further therapy. The paclitaxel arm demonstrated a 13% reduction in risk of recurrence and a 14% reduction in risk of death from disease.
    - In a similar trial by NSABP (B-28 trial),[20] AC for four cycles vs. AC for four cycles followed by pacli-

Trial	Schema		Outcome
CALGB 9344[a]	A 60 mg 75 mg 90 mg	C × 4	Paclitaxel × 4	No paclitaxel	Paclitaxel associated with a 13% reduction risk recurrence and 14% reduction risk of death
NSABP B-28[b]	AC × 4 vs AC – T Tamoxifen administered in hormone receptor-positive patients		(benefit in DFS not OS)	7% reduction in recurrence
MD Anderson[c]	FAC × 8 or paclitaxel × 4 ⟶ FAC × 4			Significant trend favoring paclitaxel
BCIRG[d]	FAC or TAC			Significant benefit from docetaxel

Figure 5-5: Role of Taxanes in Adjuvant Setting

AC, doxorubicin and cyclophosphamide; DFS, disease-free survival; FAC, 5-fluorouracil, doxorubicin, and cyclophosphamide; T, paclitaxel; TAC, docetaxel, doxorubicin, and cyclophosphamide.

[a]Henderson IC, Berry DA, Demetri GD, et al. Improved outcomes from adding sequential paclitaxel but not from escalating doxorubicin dose in an adjuvant chemotherapy regimen for patients with node-positive primary breast cancer. *J Clin Oncol.* 2003;21:976-983.

[b]Mamounas EP, Bryant J, Lembersky BC, et al. Paclitaxel (T) following doxorubicin/cyclophosphamide (AC) as adjuvant chemotherapy for node-positive breast cancer: results from NSABP B-28 [abstract]. *Proc Am Soc Clin Oncol.* 2003;22:4. Abstract 12.

[c]Valero V, Buzdar AU, McNeese M, Singletary E, Hortobagyi GN. Primary chemotherapy in the treatment of breast cancer: the University of Texas, M.D. Anderson Cancer Center experience. *Clin Breast Cancer.* 2002;(suppl 2):S63-568.

[d]Martin M, Pienkowski T, Mackey J, et al. TAC improves disease free survival over FAC in node positive early breast cancer patients, BCIRG 001, 55 months follow-up [abstract]. *Breast Cancer Res Treat.* 2003;88:43.

taxel for four cycles was associated with a 7% benefit in DFS but not in overall survival.

■ The MD Anderson Cancer Center trial of 5-fluorouracil, doxorubicin, and cyclophosphamide for eight cycles, compared with the same regimen for four cycles preceded by paclitaxel for four cycles, also demonstrated a trend favoring paclitaxel.

■ In summary, both the NSABP B-28 and CALGB 9344 trials supported the use of paclitaxel after AC for node-positive breast cancer regardless of the ER and PR status, use of tamoxifen, age of the patient, and number of positive lymph nodes. With time, this has not changed. Although all patients benefit, it is clear that patients with hormone receptor-negative breast cancer benefit to a greater degree than patients with hormone receptor-positive breast cancer.

  • Both trials were positive for DFS.
  • One trial was positive for OS (CALGB).
• All show AC → paclitaxel is superior to AC alone.
• If the Breast Cancer International Research Group (BCIRG) study is included, there is significant data to support routine taxane use.

■ Node-positive breast cancer (Table 5-11)
  • Full dose of chemotherapy is necessary
  • CMF vs. no chemotherapy has shown a benefit in terms of DFS and OS in favor of CMF.
  • EBCTCG overview (anthracycline-containing regimen vs. CMF) found a 12% further reduction in the annual odds of recurrence and a 11% further reduction in the annual odds of death with anthracycline-based treatment.
    ■ This analysis was based on 11 trials with 5,942 patients in which anthracycline-based therapy was compared with CMF. 2,157 patients in 6 trials received doxorubicin as the anthracycline and 1,320 patients received epirubicin as the anthracycline.

Table 5-11:   Axillary Node-Positive Breast Cancer: Combination Chemotherapy Options

- AC followed by paclitaxel
- FEC
- AC
- EC
- TAC
- Doxorubicin followed by CMF
- CMF alone

AC, doxorubicin and cyclophosphamide; CMF, cyclophosphamide, methotrexate, and 5-fluorouracil; EC, epirubicin and cyclophosphamide; FEC, 5-fluorouracil, epirubicin, and cyclophosphamide; TAC, docetaxel, doxorubicin, and cyclophosphamide.

- Retrospective analysis suggests superiority of anthracycline-based regimens may be limited to HER-2/neu-overexpressing breast cancer.
- Randomized trial of docetaxel, doxorubicin, cyclophosphamide (TAC) vs. 5-flourouracil, doxorubicin, cyclophosphamide (FAC) at 33 months of follow-up demonstrated that TAC was superior to FAC in patients with 1–3 positive axillary lymph nodes with respect to DFS and OS.[21] (DFS: hazard ratio [HR], 0.68; OS: HR, 0.76)
  - At 55 months of follow-up, TAC continued to demonstrate an improved DFS, with a 28% reduction in the risk of relapse and a 30% reduction in the risk of death. This benefit was irrespective of hormone receptor, node, or HER-2/neu status. Toxicity was manageable for both regimens.
    - No septic deaths
    - Greater episodes of febrile neutropenia with TAC
- Anthracycline regimens vs. CMF
  - AC for four cycles is equivalent to CMF for six cycles in terms of DFS and OS[22–27]
  - No benefit from dose intensification of doxorubicin[28,29]

- High-risk patients with four or more positive nodes demonstrated benefit from sequential therapy over alternating regimens (doxorubicin/CMF)[30]
- Randomized trial of 5-fluorouracil, epirubicin, cyclophosphamide (FEC) vs. CMF (classic) demonstrated 5-year relapse-free survival (RFS) rate of 63% vs. 53% and OS rate of 77% vs. 70% in favor of FEC[31]
  - Classic CMF: 28-day schedule, oral cyclophosphamide days 1–14; schedule of cytotoxics (methotrexate and 5-fluorouracil [5-FU]) days 1 and 8.
- In 2001, the French Adjuvant Study Group demonstrated that a higher dose of epirubicin (100 mg/m^2) was superior to 50 mg/m^2 when 5-year DFS and OS were measured.[32]
- A trial of epirubicin and cyclophosphamide (EC) low vs. high dose (50 mg/m^2 vs. 100 mg/m^2) vs. CMF showed that EC 100 mg/m^2 is equivalent to CMF in event-free survival and OS.[33]
- Adjuvant therapy dose and schedule (Figure 5-6)
  - Data demonstrate that the onset of chemotherapy may be delayed for up to 12 weeks after surgery with no adverse effect on survival.[34]
  - Dose density refers to the administration of drugs over a shortened treatment interval.
  - Dose intensity refers to the amount of drug delivered per unit of time.
  - Sequential therapy refers to the application of treatments one at a time rather than concurrently.
  - Landmark study: CALGB 9741 (Figure 5-7)
    - This was a four-arm study in which doxorubicin, cyclophosphamide, and paclitaxel were compared in an accelerated fashion (q 2 weeks) or in the standard manner (q 3 weeks) concurrently or sequentially (Table 5-12).
    - All patients had:
      - Early-stage breast cancer (T0–3, N1–2, M0)
      - Prior primary surgery
      - Adequate blood counts

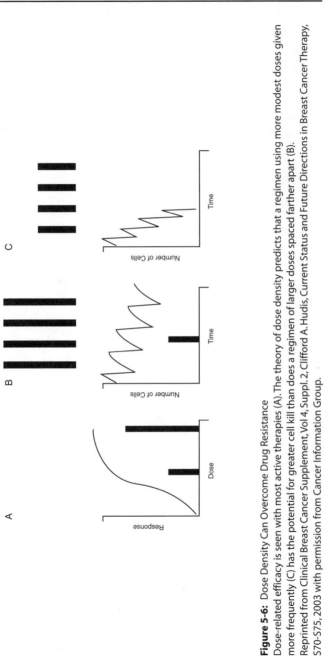

Figure 5-6: Dose Density Can Overcome Drug Resistance

Dose-related efficacy is seen with most active therapies (A). The theory of dose density predicts that a regimen using more modest doses given more frequently (C) has the potential for greater cell kill than does a regimen of larger doses spaced farther apart (B). Reprinted from Clinical Breast Cancer Supplement, Vol 4, Suppl. 2, Clifford A. Hudis, Current Status and Future Directions in Breast Cancer Therapy, S70–S75, 2003 with permission from Cancer Information Group.

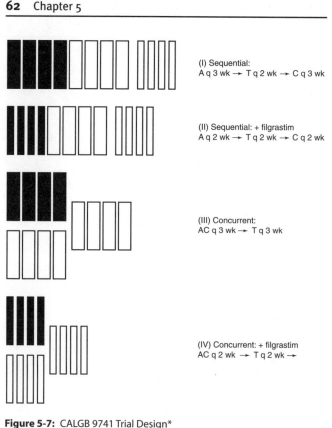

Figure 5-7: CALGB 9741 Trial Design*
Doses: A = 60 mg/m^2, T = 175 mg/m^2, and C = 600 mg/^{2}.
A, doxorubicin; C, cyclophosphamide; T, paclitaxel.
Citron M, et al. Randomized trial of dose-dense vs. conventionally scheduled and sequential versus concurrent combination chemotherapy as postoperative adjuvant treatment of node positive primary breast cancer: first report of Intergroup Trial C9741/Cancer and Leukemia Group B Trial 9741. *J CO.* 2003;21:1431-1439.

- Normal chest x-ray and EKG
- 988 patients in the 2-week schedule (493 sequential q 2 weeks, 495 concurrent q 2 weeks)
- 989 patients in the 3-week regimen (488 sequential q 3 weeks, 501 concurrent q 3 weeks)

Table 5-12:   Treatment Intervals: Dose-Dense Therapy

Study	Trial design	Outcome
CALGB 9741[a]	AC–T Sequential vs. concurrent Every 3 wk vs. every 2 wk	Dose-dense treatment associated with a 26% proportional reduction in 4-yr DFS (82% for dose-dense and 75% for every-3-week regimens) ($P = 0.010$)
SWOG[b]	CMFVP (52 wk) vs. FAC-M (20 wk)	No demonstration of superiority with doxorubicin regimen
Venturini[c]	FEC std interval q 3 wk vs. Accelerated q 2 wk with GCSF day 4–11	No difference in RFS Trend longer survival in dose-dense arm

AC, doxorubicin and cyclophosphamide; CMFVP, cyclophosphamide, methotrexate, 5-fluorouracil, vincristine, and prednisone; FAC-M, 5-fluorouracil, doxorubicin, cyclophosphamide, and methotrexate; FEC, 5-fluorouracil, epirubicin, and cyclophosphamide; GCSF, granulocyte colony-stimulating factor; T, paclitaxel.

[a]Citron M, Berry DA, Cirrincione C, et al. Superiority of dose-dense (DD) over conventional scheduling (CS) and equivalence of sequential (SC) vs combination adjuvant chemotherapy (CC) for node positive breast cancer (CALGB 9741, INT C9741) [abstract]. *Breast Cancer Res Treat.* 2002;76(suppl 1):A-15.

[b]Bonadonna G, Valagussa P, Rossi A. Ten-year experience with CMF-based adjuvant chemotherapy in resectable breast cancer. *Breast Cancer Res Treat.* 1985;5:95-115.

[c]Venturini M, Aitini E, Del Mastro L, et al. Phase III adjuvant trial comparing standard vs accelerated FEC regimen in early breast cancer patients. Results from GONO-M1G1 study [abstract]. *Breast Cancer Res Treat.* 2003;82(suppl 1):59. Abstract 12.

- Superior survival in the group receiving therapy every 2 weeks (dose-dense schedule)
  - At a median of 36 months follow-up, the dose-dense treatment was associated with a 26% proportional reduction in relapse ($P=0.010$). The 4-year DFS rate was 82% for dose-dense schedule and 75% for the every-3-week regimens.
  - The secondary end point of this trial was OS. The dose-dense treatment was associated with a 31% proportional reduction in mortality ($P=0.013$). The 3-year OS rate was 92% in the dose-dense schedule and 90% in the every-3-week schedule.
  - Toxicities for both regimens were acceptable and grade 4 granulocytopenia, defined as an absolute neutrophil count of less than 500 cells/mm^3, was more frequent with the 3-week schedule, presumably secondary to the use of growth factors with the 2-week regimen. This trial also confirmed a baseline absolute neutrophil count of 1,000 cells/mm^3 is safe for the administration of cytotoxic chemotherapy.
- Two other randomized studies show support for dose-dense therapy (see Table 5-12).
- High-dose chemotherapy with autograft support
  - To date, no study has demonstrated a beneficial effect. This still remains an area for clinical investigations with different approaches.[35]
- Adjuvant chemotherapy for node-negative breast cancer
  - Because of a demonstrated benefit, polychemotherapy should be considered in patients with early-stage breast cancer regardless of:
    - Node status
    - Hormone receptor status
    - Menopausal status
  - Polychemotherapy's effect is independent of the benefits from endocrine treatment.
  - Historically, the CMF regimen has been considered the standard of care in node-negative disease.

Table 5-13:   Axillary Node-Negative Breast Cancer: Combination Chemotherapy Options

- Cyclophosphamide, methotrexate, 5-flourouracil (CMF)
- Cyclophosphamide, doxorubicin, 5-flourouracil (CAF/FAC)
- Doxorubicin and cyclophosphamide (AC)

- Several other combinations are also alternatively used (Table 5-13).
- Most regimens are well tolerated.
- In general, however, the following should be considered for each individual patient:
  - Life expectancy
  - Comorbid conditions
  - Patient desires and expectations
- Treatment benefits vs. toxicities and patient expectations must be considered.
- The major validated indication for chemotherapy in node-negative disease is tumor size, especially in tumors that are also hormone receptor-negative. It is generally accepted that a discussion regarding treatment with chemotherapy should be initiated with patients having a tumor 1 cm or larger, even with negative nodes.
- St. Gallen International Consensus Panel[36] identified unfavorable prognostic factors (Table 5-14).
- In node-negative disease with small tumors, absolute benefit from chemotherapy may be small. Therefore, it is important to estimate prognosis.
- Tools available to help
  - AdjuvantOnline software program[37] (Table 5-15)

Table 5-14:   Node-Negative Breast Cancer: Unfavorable Prognostic Factors

- Negative hormone receptors
- Pathologic tumor size greater than 2 cm
- Histologic and/or nuclear grade 2–3
- Age less than 35 years

Table 5-15:   AdjuvantOnline

- Estimates derived from SEER tumor registry database
- Contains data on 2,000 HR-negative
                      9,000 HR-positive Node-negative patients
- Estimates breast cancer-related mortality (directly derived from SEER data)
- Estimates relapse rate (indirectly derived from SEER data)
- Defines relapse: local regional relapse
                    distant relapse
                    contralateral relapse
- Includes more accurate mortality rates
- Has been updated to include treatment with aromatase inhibitors as well as dose-dense therapy with CMF

HR, hormone receptor; SEER, Surveillance Epidemiology and End Results.

- Available on-line and takes into account:
  - Patient's age
  - Comorbid conditions
  - Estrogen receptor status
  - Tumor grade
  - Tumor size
  - Number of positive nodes
- Calculates risk for relapse as well as mortality and considers both hormonal therapy and chemotherapy
- Validated when compared with a large cooperative group study (NSABP B-20 and B-14)
- NSABP study[39]
- FinProg Study[40]—Web-based nationwide breast cancer database
- Gene microarray technology is a future tool designed to permit evaluation based on a molecular profile as opposed to a single feature (eg, tumor size).
- Adjuvant therapy for HER-2/neu-overexpressing breast cancer
  - Currently there are two adjuvant trials exploring 52 weeks of trastuzumab in combination with taxanes,

anthracyclines, and cyclophosphamide regimens in various schedules (Figure 5-8) and one randomized trial exploring 1 or 2 years of trastuzumab following primary therapy (chemotherapy +/− radiation—the Herceptin Adjuvant [HERA] Trial).

- Two of the trials, NSABP B-31 and the NCCTG N9831 Intergroup trial, were recently presented as part of a first interim analysis.[38] Although the schedules were slightly different regarding paclitaxel administration (175 mg/m^2 every 3 weeks vs. 80 mg/m^2 weekly for 12 weeks), trastuzumab was administered in a standard fashion. These studies were presented as a combined analysis of doxorubicin and cyclophosphamide followed by paclitaxel with or without trastuzumab. The median follow-up was 2 years. Primary and secondary end points

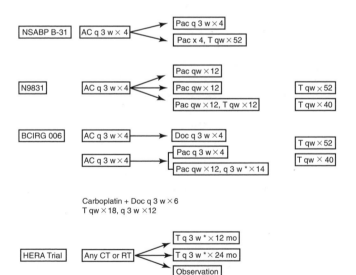

Figure 5-8: Summary of Ongoing Trastuzumab Adjuvant Therapy Trials*
*q 3 w at 6 mg/kg.
AC, doxorubicin and cyclophosphamide; CT, chemotherapy; Doc, docetaxel; Pac, paclitaxel; RT, radiotherapy; T, trastuzumab.
Horton J. HER2 and trastuzumab in breast cancer. *Cancer Control.* 2001;8:103–110.

were DFS, OS, and time to first distant recurrence, respectively. The initial findings of this analysis demonstrated that when trastuzumab is given concurrently with paclitaxel following AC chemotherapy, the risk of a first breast cancer event at 3 years is reduced by 52%. It was also noted that the addition of trastuzumab reduced the probability of distant recurrence by 53% at 3 years and that the hazard of developing distant metastases decreased over time.

- The HERA trial, a European multi-institution trial, in which patients are randomized to trastuzumab at 3-week intervals for 12 or 24 months vs. observation, had interim results of the 1-year arm presented at the May 2005 meeting of the American Society of Clinical Oncology (ASCO). These findings support the use of trastuzumab in the adjuvant setting following primary therapy for breast cancer. At a median 1-year follow-up, trastuzumab administered on an every-3-week schedule to women with HER-2/neu-positive breast cancer following adjuvant chemotherapy prolonged the disease-free and relapse-free survival (2-year DFS, 85% with trastuzumab vs. 77.4% with observation [HR, 0.54; $P < 0.0001$]). Trastuzumab also was found to significantly reduce the risk of distant metastases (of 220 patients in the observation arm—154 had a distant metastatic event. Of the 127 in the treatment arm of 1-yr trastuzumab 85 patients had a distant event). Of note, these benefits were reported to be independent of the baseline characteristics of the tumor (eg, node status, hormone receptor status, the type of adjuvant therapy received). Also of note, in this trial the incidence of severe symptomatic congestive heart failure was low (0.5%).

- Multiple gated acquisition (MUGA) scans should be obtained prior to starting treatment, 8 weeks after treatment, and then at the clinician's discretion.

  - An interim cardiac safety analysis of the NCCTG N9831 Intergroup adjuvant trial was presented at the May 2005 ASCO Meeting.[41] In this 3-arm, randomized phase III trial, patients received AC standard doses at 3-week intervals (doxorubicin 60 mg/m^2, cyclophosphamide 600 mg/m^2), followed by weekly paclitaxel 80 mg/m^2 for 12 weeks either alone [arm A], followed by trastuzumab at standard doses [arm B], or concurrently with trastuzumab [arm C]. Trastuzumab was continued for 1 year. Left ventricular ejection fraction was evaluated by MUGA scan or echocardiography (ECHO) at set intervals (pretherapy, and 3, 6, 9, and 18 months following registration). The study enrolled 3,505 patients. The study accrual was completed on April 29, 2005. In analyzing the separate arms, there were no cardiovascular events in arm A (nontrastuzumab), and 13 events (2.2%) in arm B (trastuzumab following paclitaxel), and 20 events (3.3%) in arm C (concurrent trastuzumab and paclitaxel) (Table 5-16).

- Stage III invasive breast cancer (T_3, N_1, M_0)
  - Important to do staging work-up:
    - Bone scan
    - CT (chest, abdomen, and pelvis)
  - Postsurgical adjuvant therapy is similar to what is administered for stage II disease.

Table 5-16:   Cardiac Toxicity Herceptin Adjuvant Trial N9831

	No. of events	Percentage	Event
Arm A	0	0	
Arm B	13	2.2%	12–CHF 1–Cardiac arrest 6 yrs post trial entry
Arm C	20	3.3%	19–CHF 1–Cardiac failure 8 mos. post trial entry

70 Chapter 5

■ References

1. Early Breast Cancer Trialists' Collaborative Group. Tamoxifen for early breast cancer: an overview of the randomised trials. *Lancet.* 1998;351:1451-1467.
2. NIH Consensus Development Program O. Consensus Statements: Adjuvant therapy for breast cancer. In: NIH Consensus Development Conference; 2000. http://consensus.nih.gov/2000/2000adjuvanttherapybreastcancer114html.htm
3. Early Breast Cancer Trialists' Collaborative Group. Effects of chemotherapy and hormonal therapy for early breast cancer on recurrence and a 15-year survival: an overview of the randomised trials. *Lancet.* 2005;365:1687-1717.
4. Elledge RM, Green S, Pugh R, et al. Estrogen receptor (ER) and progesterone receptor (PgR), by ligand-binding assay compared with ER, PgR and pS2, by immunohistochemistry in predicting response to tamoxifen in metastatic breast cancer: a Southwest Oncology Group Study. *Int J Cancer.* 2000;89:111-117.
5. Lake DE, Hudis C. Aromatase inhibitors in breast cancer: an update. *Cancer Control.* 2002;9:490-498.
6. Leonard RC. Adjuvant therapy for premenopausal and postmenopausal women. In: *2004 Educational Book.* American Society of Clinical Oncology; 2004:3.
7. Early Breast Cancer Trialists' Collaborative Group. Ovarian ablation in early breast cancer: overview of the randomized trials. *Lancet.* 1996;348:1189-1196.
8. Gull B, Karlsson B, Milsom I, Granberg S. Can ultrasound replace dilation and curettage? A longitudinal evaluation of postmenopausal bleeding and transvaginal sonographic measurement of the endometrium as predictors of endometrial cancer. *Am J Obstet Gynecol.* 2003;188:401-408.
9. Baum M, Budzar AU, Cuzick J, et al. Anastrozole alone or in combination with tamoxifen versus tamoxifen alone for adjuvant treatment of postmenopausal women with early breast cancer: first results of the ATAC randomised trial. *Lancet.* 2002;359:2131-2139.
10. Baum M, Buzdar A, Cuzick J, et al. Anastrozole alone or in combination with tamoxifen versus tamoxifen alone for adjuvant treatment of postmenopausal women with early-stage breast cancer: results of the ATAC (Arimidex, Tamoxifen Alone or in Combination) trial efficacy and safety update analyses. *Cancer.* 2003;98:1802-1810.

11. Goss PE, Ingle JN, Martino S, et al. A randomized trial of letrozole in postmenopausal women after five years of tamoxifen therapy for early-stage breast cancer. *N Engl J Med.* 2003;349:1793-1802.

12. Howell A, on behalf of the ATAC Trialists Group. Effect of anastrozole on bone mineral density: 2-year results of the arimidex (anastrozole), tamoxifen, alone or in combination (ATAC) trial [abstract]. *Breast Cancer Res Treat.* 2003; 82(suppl 1):S27. Abstract 129.

13. Lonning PE, Geisler J, Krag LE, et al. Effect of exemestane on bone: a randomized placebo controlled study in post-menopausal women with early breast cancer at low risk. In: *2004 American Society of Clinical Oncology Annual Meeting Proceedings* (Post-Meeting Edition). 2004;22:518.

14. Sawada S, Sato K. Effect of anastrozole and tamoxifen on serum lipids levels in Japanese postmenopausal women with early breast cancer [abstract]. *Breast Cancer Res Treat.* 2003;88:S31-S32.

15. Rose C, Vtoraya O, Pluzanska A, et al. An open randomised trial of second-line endocrine therapy in advanced breast cancer. Comparison of the aromatase inhibitors letrozole and anastrozole. *Eur J Cancer.* 2003;39:2318-2327.

16. Early Breast Cancer Trialists' Collaborative Group. Polychemotherapy for early breast cancer: an overview of the randomized trials. *Lancet.* 1998;352:930-942.

17. Goldhirsch A, Wood WC, Gelber RD, Coates AS, Thurlimann B, Senn HJ. Meeting highlights: updated international expert consensus on the primary therapy of early breast cancer. *J Clin Oncol.* 2003;21:3357-3365.

18. Early Breast Cancer Trialists' Collaborative Group. Systemic treatment of early breast cancer by hormonal, cytotoxic, or immune therapy. 133 randomised trials involving 31,000 recurrences and 24,000 deaths among 75,000 women. *Lancet.* 1992;339:71-85.

19. Henderson IC, Berry DA, Demetri GD, et al. Improved outcomes from adding sequential Paclitaxel but not from escalating doxorubicin dose in an adjuvant chemotherapy regimen for patients with node-positive primary breast cancer. *J Clin Oncol.* 2003;21:976-983.

20. Mamounas EP, Bryant J, Lembersky BC, et al. Paclitaxel (T) following doxorubicin/cyclophosphamide (AC) as adjuvant chemotherapy for node-positive breast cancer: results from NSABP B-28 [abstract]. *Proc Am Soc Clin Oncol.* 2003;22:4. Abstract 12.

21. Martin M, Pienkowski T, Mackey J, et al. TAC improves disease free survival and overall survival over FAC in node positive early breast cancer patients, BCIRG 001, 55 months follow-up. Abstract presented at: San Antonio BRCA Symposium; December 5, 2003; San Antonio, TX.

22. Bang SM, Heo DS, Lee KH, et al. Adjuvant doxorubicin and cyclophosphamide versus cyclophosphamide, methotrexate, and 5-fluorouracil chemotherapy in premenopausal women with axillary lymph node positive breast carcinoma. *Cancer.* 2000;89:2521-2526.

23. Fisher B, Anderson S, Tan-Chiu E, et al. Tamoxifen and chemotherapy for axillary node-negative, estrogen receptor-negative breast cancer: findings from National Surgical Adjuvant Breast and Bowel Project B-23. *J Clin Oncol.* 2001;19:931-942.

24. Fisher B, Brown AM, Dimitrov NV, et al. Two months of doxorubicin-cyclophosphamide with and without interval reinduction therapy compared with 6 months of cyclophosphamide, methotrexate, and fluorouracil in positive-node breast cancer patients with tamoxifen-nonresponsive tumors: results from the National Surgical Breast and Bowel Project B-15. *J Clin Oncol.* 1990;8:1483-1496.

25. Seidman A, Hudis C, Pierri MK, et al. Cardiac dysfunction in the trastuzumab clinical trials experience. *J Clin Oncol.* 2002;20:1215-1221.

26. Theodoulou M, Seidman AD. Cardiac effects of adjuvant therapy for early breast cancer. *Semin Oncol.* 2003;30:730-739.

27. Valero V, Perez E, Dieras V. Doxorubicin and taxane combination regimens for metastatic breast cancer: focus on cardiac effects. *Semin Oncol.* 2001;28(suppl 12):15-23.

28. Perez EA. Doxorubicin and paclitaxel in the treatment of advanced breast cancer: efficacy and cardiac considerations. *Cancer Invest.* 2001;19:155-164.

29. Henderson IC, Berry D, Demetri G, et al. Improved disease-free (DFS) and overall survival (OS) from the addition of sequential paclitaxel (T) but not from the escalation of doxorubicin (A) dose level in the adjuvant chemotherapy of patients (pts) with node-positive primary breast cancer (BC) [abstract]. *Proc Am Soc Clin Oncol.* 1998;17:101A:390A. Abstract 390.

30. Bonadonna G, Zambetti M, Valagussa P. Sequential or alternating doxorubicin and CMF regimens in breast cancer with

more than three positive nodes. Ten-year results. *JAMA.* 1995;273:542-547.

31. Levine MN, Bramwell VH, Pritchard KI, et al. Randomized trial of intensive cyclophosphamide, epirubicin, and fluorouracil chemotherapy compared with cyclophosphamide, methotrexate, and fluorouracil in premenopausal women with node-positive breast cancer. *J Clin Oncol.* 1998; 16:2651-2658.

32. French Adjuvant Study Group. Benefit of a high-dose epirubicin regimen in adjuvant chemotherapy for node-positive breast cancer patients with poor prognostic factors: 5-year follow-up results of French Adjuvant Study Group 05 randomized trial. *J Clin Oncol.* 2001;19:602-611.

33. Piccart MJ, Di Leo A, Beauduin M, et al. Phase III trial comparing two dose levels of epirubicin combined with cyclophosphamide with cyclophosphamide, methotrexate, and fluorouracil in node-positive breast cancer. *J Clin Oncol.* 2001;19:3103-3110.

34. Lohrisch C, Gelmon K, Paltiel C, et al. Delivery of adjuvant chemotherapy for breast cancer more than 12 weeks after definitive surgery may compromise survival [abstract]. *Breast Cancer Res Treat.* 2003;88:S27. Abstract 130.

35. Lake DE, Hudis CA. High-dose chemotherapy in breast cancer. *Drugs.* 2004;64:1851-1860.

36. Goldhirsch A, Wood WC, Gelber RD, Coates AS, Thurlimann B, Senn HJ. Meeting highlights: updated international expert consensus on the primary therapy of early breast cancer. *J Clin Oncol.* 2003;21:3357-3365.

37. Adjuvant! Inc. AdjuvantOnline [Web site]. Available at: http://adjuvantonline.com/index1.html. Accessed June 1, 2005.

38. Romond EH, Perez E, Bryant J, Suman V, et al. Doxorubicin & cyclophosphamide followed by paclitaxel with or without trastuzumab as adjuvant therapy for patients with HER2-positive operable breast cancer: combined analysis of NSABP-B31/NCCTG N9831. In press. Paper presented at: Annual Meeting of American Society of Clinical Oncology; May 15, 2005; Orlando, FL.

39. Fisher B, Dignam J, Tan-Chiu E, et al. Prognosis and treatment of patients with breast tumors of one centimeter or less and negative axillary lymph nodes. *J Natl Cancer Inst.* 2001;93:112-120.

40.   The FinProg Research Group. The Finprog Study: a Nationwide Breast Cancer Database [Web site]. Available at: http://www.finprog.org. Accessed June 1, 2005.

41.   Perez E, Suman V, Davidson N, et al. Interim cardiac safety anaylsis of NCCTG N9831 Intergroup adjuvant trastuzumab trial. *J Clin Oncol*. 2005;23(suppl):17s.

CHAPTER 6

Neoadjuvant Therapy

■ Rationale for Neoadjuvant Therapy

■ Ten percent to 30% of all primary breast cancers are locally advanced.
■ Defined as first postdiagnosis systemic treatment
■ Who should be treated in neoadjuvant fashion?
  ● Most cases of stage IIIA or T3–4 disease including:
    ■ Inflammatory breast cancer
    ■ Patients with positive ipsilateral supraclavicular or infraclavicular nodes

■ Objectives of Neoadjuvant Therapy

■ Decrease spread of metastatic disease
■ Reduce the size of an initially unresectable tumor (in an attempt to allow for breast-conserving surgery [BCS])
■ Improve local control
■ Provide an opportunity for testing novel therapies and biomarkers, and for investigating molecular profiling

■ Principles Addressed in Randomized Trials

■ In general, treatment is similar to that of early-stage disease.

■ Conclusions of Multiple Randomized Trials

■ Neoadjuvant chemotherapy is a safe option for the treatment of operable breast cancer.
  ● May aid in the estimate of prognosis and choice of appropriate adjuvant chemotherapy

- With a median time on study of 1.8–8 months NSABP B27 trial has demonstrated taxane therapy is of additional benefit.
  - Pathological response was greatest in the group with preop taxane plus AC.
  - Fewer local recurrences occurred in the taxane arms.
- Pending further maturation additional survival information will be provided.
- Taxane therapy is clearly of additional benefit in terms of response
  - Can convert nonresponders to responders
  - The role of concurrent vs. sequential therapy is unclear, but current data favors sequential.
  - Administration every 3 weeks vs. weekly is being studied.
  - The majority of data is with docetaxel.
    - Appears relatively well tolerated, with the following side effects:
      - Radiation recall reactions
      - Musculoskeletal symptoms
- No survival benefit with neoadjuvant therapy

■ New Directions in Neoadjuvant Treatment of Breast Cancer

- Use of improved imaging techniques to predict response and prognosis, and to improve understanding of the local extent of disease
  - ACRIN-MRI national neoadjuvant trial
- Serial biopsies to determine molecular predictors of response to therapy
  - Multiple studies ongoing
- Prospective allocation of treatment based on molecular profiling
- Changing chemotherapy sequence and schedule to improve response to therapy
- Neoadjuvant hormonal therapy for elderly or impaired patients

CHAPTER 7

Radiation for Early-Stage Disease

■ Rationale for Radiation for Early Breast Cancer

■ To reduce risk of local recurrence

■ Indications[1]

■ All cases of breast-conserving therapy
■ Postmastectomy with a primary tumor greater than or equal to 5 cm
■ Four or more positive lymph nodes
■ May not be necessary in patients older than 70 years of age with hormone receptor-positive tumors less than 2 cm if given tamoxifen[2]

■ Schedule

■ Majority of randomized trials reported results based on
   • 40–54 cGy in 16–27 fractions
   • Some also used a boost of 600 cGy radiation to the primary site (surgical bed).
■ Effectiveness is similar for different approaches.

■ Accelerated Radiotherapy

■ Defined as a large daily dose of radiation administered in a shorter period of time
■ Total dose is usually less to avoid toxicity.
■ Several randomized studies showed no difference in local recurrence rates.
■ The Institute of Cancer Research (ICR) showed less skin changes with accelerated fractions.
■ Possible contraindications

- Breast tissue greater than 25 cm in thickness at mid-point of radiation field
- Margins not rendered clear after BCS
- Toxicity concerns
  - Cardiac
  - Pneumonitis

■ Boost Irradiation

- Defined as additional radiation to the surgical bed
- Rationale for use
  - Most local recurrences occur in the surgical bed; therefore, a higher dose in this area should reduce risk.
- Differences between whole breast and boost irradiation radiotherapy
  - Whole breast radiotherapy is delivered by two tangential parallel fields to the chest wall.
  - Boost irradiation
    - Follows whole breast treatment
    - Delivered with a single direct field
    - Uses electron therapy
- Three trials[3–5] showed no survival benefit for those receiving boost radiation.
- Increased cosmetic morbidity was noted in those receiving boost technique radiation therapy.
- Patients who received greatest benefit
  - Those aged less than 50 years
  - Those with a higher risk of local recurrence

■ Regional Lymph Node Irradiation Rationale (Tables 7-1 and 7-2)

- Risk of regional recurrence 10 years after anthracycline chemotherapy with or without endocrine treatment:[6]
  - 4% in patients with 1–3 positive lymph nodes
  - 6% in patients with 4–9 positive lymph nodes
- Objective is to sterilize the nodes and intransit metastases to prevent locoregional recurrence.
- Locoregional radiation can reduce distant recurrences.

Table 7-1: Unanswered Locoregional Radiotherapy Questions

- Appropriate to use in patients with 1–3 positive axillary nodes?
- Which regional nodes to include in radiotherapy field?
  - Axillary
  - Internal mammary
  - Both
- Should patients receiving BCS and WBRT receive additional nodal irradiation?

BCS, breast-conserving therapy; WBRT, whole breast radiation therapy.

- ASCO guidelines
  - Postmastectomy patients at high risk for local recurrence receive locoregional radiation.
    - Primary tumor > 5 cm
    - Four or more positive lymph nodes in the axilla
- Ongoing trials address the issue of additional nodal irradiation after BCS and the need to include internal mammary nodes.[7,8]

■ New Radiation Therapy Techniques Under Evaluation

- Accelerated partial breast radiotherapy
- Intensity modulated radiation therapy (IMRT) to the breast/chest wall and regional lymph nodes

Table 7-2: Toxicities Associated with Regional Radiotherapy

- Lymphedema
- Pneumonitis
- Cardiac disease
- Second malignancies
  - Leukemia
  - Solid tumors (esophageal, lung)

■ References

1. Recht A, Edge SB, Solin LJ, et al. Postmastectomy radio-therapy: clinical practice guidelines of the American Society of Clinical Oncology. *J Clin Oncol.* 2001;19:1539-1569.

2. Smith IE, Ross GM. Breast radiotherapy after lumpectomy—no longer always necessary. *N Engl J Med.* 2004; 351:1021-1023.

3. Bartelink H, Horiot JC, Poortmans P, et al. Recurrence rates after treatment of breast cancer with standard radiotherapy with or without additional radiation. *N Engl J Med.* 2001; 345:1378-1387.

4. Romestaing P, Lehingue Y, Carrie C, et al. Role of a 10-Gy boost in the conservative treatment of early breast cancer: results of a randomized clinical trial in Lyon, France. *J Clin Oncol.* 1997;15:963-968.

5. Teissier E, Hery M, Ramaioli A, et al. Boost in conservative treatment 6 years results of randomized trial [abstract]. *Breast Cancer Res Treat.* 1998;50:287. Abstract 345.

6. Taghian AG, Bryant J, Anderson S, et al. Pattern of regional failure in patients with breast cancer treated by lumpectomy, breast radiation +/- chemotherapy and/or tamoxifen with no regional radiation: results from 10 NSABP randomized trials. *Int J Radiat Oncol Biol Phys.* 2003;50:S168.

7. Olivotto IA, Chua B, Elliott EA, et al. A clinical trial of breast radiation therapy versus breast plus regional radiation therapy in early-stage breast cancer: the MA20 trial. *Clin Breast Cancer.* 2003;4:361-363.

8. Poortmans P, Kouloulias VE, Venselaar JL, et al. Quality assurance of EORTC trial 22922/10925 investigating the role of internal mammary–medial supraclavicular irradiation in stage I–III breast cancer: the individual case review. *Eur J Cancer.* 2003;39:2035-2042.

CHAPTER 8

Management Issues in Metastatic Breast Cancer

■ Metastatic Breast Cancer (MBC) Management Overview

- Choice of therapeutic options depends on multiple variables (Table 8-1).
- MBC is considered a chronic illness.
- Goals of management are control of disease and maintenance of quality of life.
- Initial evaluation
  - Complete history
  - Complete physical examination
  - Pathologic documentation of stage IV breast cancer should be attempted, except when a biopsy poses a risk and the clinical picture is characteristic.
  - If possible confirm (reconfirm) hormone receptor and HER-2/neu status.
  - Baseline laboratory evaluation should include:
    - CBC
    - Comprehensive biochemical profile
    - Tumor markers: CEA and CA15-3 or BRCA 27:29
  - Pretreatment radionuclide heart scan (MUGA) if a cardiotoxic agent is being administered
  - Radiographics: bone scan; CT of chest, abdomen, and pelvis
  - MRI or CT of brain should be performed only if clinically indicated.
- General approach to patient
  - Use of sequential hormonal therapies whenever possible
  - Use of trastuzumab when indicated for HER-2/neu-overexpressing tumors

Table 8-1: Variables to Consider in Choosing Options for Management of Metastatic Breast Cancer

- Menopausal status
- Hormone receptor status
- HER-2/neu status
- Interval from prior adjuvant therapy or previous regimen for MBC
- Patient age
- Comorbid conditions
- Tumor burden and sites of disease

MBC, metastatic breast cancer.

- Use of sequential single chemotherapeutic agents or combination therapy regimens
- Indications for chemotherapy
  - Hormone receptor-negative disease
  - Patients with a visceral crisis or rapidly progressing disease
  - Patients with a high tumor burden
- Chemotherapy approaches in MBC (Tables 8-2 and 8-3)
  - Goals to keep in mind include palliation of disease, maintenance of quality of life, and survival.
  - In general, treatment with sequential single agents yields survival similar to treatment with combination regimens but with a better quality of life (Table 8-4).

Table 8-2: Single Agents Active in Metastatic Breast Cancer

- Taxanes (docetaxel, paclitaxel, nanoparticle albumin paclitaxel)
- Anthracyclines (doxorubicin, epirubicin)
- Liposomal anthracyclines (liposomal doxorubicin, liposomal daunorubicin)
- Alkylating agents (cyclophosphamide)
- Antimetabolites (methotrexate)
- Fluoropyrimidines (capecitabine, 5-fluorouracil)
- Vinca alkaloids (vinorelbine)
- Targeted agents (trastuzumab)
- Others (gemcitabine, carboplatin, etoposide, irinotecan)

Table 8-3:   Combination Agents Frequently Used in Metastatic Breast Cancer

- Anthracycline based
    - CAF
    - FEC
    - AT or A/docetaxel
- CMF
- Newer doublets
    - Docetaxel/capecitabine
    - Paclitaxel/gemcitabine
    - Carboplatin/taxane +/− trastuzumab

AT, doxorubicin and paclitaxel; CAF, cyclophosphamide, doxorubicin, and 5-fluorouracil; CMF, cyclophosphamide, epirubicin, and cyclophosphamide; FEC, 5-fluorouracil, epirubicin, and cyclophosphamide.

- Responses may be more rapid with combination agents.
- If a rapid response is not required, monotherapy should be considered first. If the patient has received prior anthracycline/taxane treatment in the adjuvant setting, capecitabine can be considered. For patients

Table 8-4:   Single Agents for Metastatic Breast Cancer Under Investigation

Antifols
Pemetrexed

Antitubulins
Epothilones

Platinum compounds
Carboplatinum

Taxanes
Nanoparticle albumin-bound paclitaxel*

*Not associated with hypersensitivity reactions, requires no premedication with steroids, and has a high therapeutic index.

without prior taxane treatment, starting with docetaxel or paclitaxel should be considered. (Note: docetaxel every 3 weeks and weekly paclitaxel are more effective than paclitaxel every 3 weeks)

- HER-2/neu-positive MBC
  - The pivotal trial to document a DFS benefit in MBC from trastuzumab combined with chemotherapy was first reported by Slamon and colleagues[1] (Figure 8-1).
  - There is documented survival benefit whenever trastuzumab is combined with chemotherapy.
  - Therefore, in the setting of MBC, trastuzumab in combination with a chemotherapy agent should be considered. Trastuzumab demonstrates synergistic or additive effects when used in combination with many agents (Table 8-5).
  - First-line therapy in HER-2/neu-positive MBC should be a taxane combined with trastuzumab. The results of the M77001 trial suggest that docetaxel may be the preferred taxane.[2]
    - This was a randomized trial between docetaxel 100 mg/m^2 every 3 weeks and docetaxel plus trastuzumab standard dose. The objective response

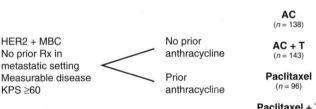

Figure 8-1: Phase III Trial of Trastuzumab in Combination with Chemotherapy: First-Line Therapy
KPS, Karnofsky Performance Status; MBC, metastatic breast cancer.
Slamon DJ, Leyland-Jones B, Shak S, et al. Use of chemotherapy plus a monoclonal antibody against HER2 for metastatic breast cancer that over-expresses HER2. *N Engl J Med.* 2001;344:783-792.

Table 8-5:   Trastuzumab and Chemotherapy: In Vitro Cytotoxicity Against HER-2/neu-Positive Breast Cancer Cell Lines[a–d]

Synergistic (CI<1)		Additive (CI~1)		Subadditive (CI>1)	
Vinorelbine	0.34	Doxorubicin	0.82-1.16	5-Fluorouracil	2.87
Docetaxel/ carboplatin	0.34	Paclitaxel	0.91		
Docetaxel	0.41	Epirubicin	0.99		
Etoposide	0.54	Vinblastine	1.09		
Cyclophosphamide	0.57	Methotrexate	1.36		
Paclitaxel/ carboplatin	0.64				
Thiotepa	0.67				
Cisplatin	0.67				
Liposomal doxorubicin	0.7				
Gemcitabine	<0.5–>5 (variable, dose-dependent)				

*Based on a combination index (CI) score from multiple drug-effect analysis at fixed molar ratios.

[a]Pegram M, Hsu S, Lewis G, et al. Inhibitory effects of combinations of HER-2/neu antibody and chemotherapeutic agents used for treatment of human breast cancers. *Oncogene.* 1999:18:2241-2251.

[b]Pegram MD, Lopez A, Konecny G, Slamon DJ. Trastuzumab and chemotherapeutics: drug interactions and synergies. *Semin Oncol.* 2000;27(suppl 11):21-25; discussion 92-100.

[c]Nabholtz JM, Slamon D. New adjuvant strategies for breast cancer: meeting the challenge of intergrating chemotherapy and trastuzumab (Herceptin). *Semin Oncol.* 28(suppl 3):1-12.

[d]Hirsch FR, Helfrich B, Franklin Wa, Varella-Garcia M, Chan DC, Bunn PA Jr. Preclinical studies of gemcitabine and trastuzumab in breast and lung cancer cell lines. *Clin Breast Cancer.* 2002;3(suppl 1):12-16.

rate was significantly higher for the docetaxel–trastuzumab group (61% vs. 34%, $P=0.0002$). The combined therapy arm also demonstrated an increase in the median duration of response (11.7 vs. 5.7 mo) as well as the time to progression (11.7 vs. 6.1 mo).[3]

- An unresolved question is how long trastuzumab should be used in the face of disease progression.
- The patient's extent of disease, performance status, and comorbid conditions should still be considered. Patients with bone-only disease and/or minimal tumor burden that is hormone receptor-positive and HER-2/neu-overexpressing may still be offered hormonal therapy. Studies favor using an aromatase inhibitor over tamoxifen in these patients with HER-2/neu-positive disease.
- Weekly or 3-week infusion schedule of trastuzumab demonstrates similar results (Table 8-6).
- Chemotherapy is not without toxicities and hypersensitivity reactions. Commonly reported reactions are listed in Table 8-7.

■ Hormonal therapy in MBC
  - Numerous options include tamoxifen, aromatase inhibitors, SERDs (fulvestrant), and second-generation agents such as megestrol, androgens, and estrogens.
  - Menopausal status should be considered in making decision (Table 8-8).
  - Leuprolide 7.5 mg or goserelin acetate 3.8 mg may be administered monthly through a deep subcutaneous injection to render a premenopausal patient postmenopausal.

Table 8-6:   Trastuzumab Dosing

	Weekly	Every 3 weeks
Initial dose (loading)	4 mg/kg × 1	8 mg/kg × 1
Subsequent dose	2 mg/kg × 1 week	6 mg/kg every 3 weeks

- The optimal sequencing of endocrine therapies is yet to be defined. If a patient has received tamoxifen in the adjuvant setting and experiences progression of metastases, an aromatase inhibitor should be considered. Upon further progression a SERD (eg, fulvestrant) should be considered. If there has been a long interval from the last tamoxifen use, tamoxifen can be used again. When MBC is refractory to newer agents, megestrol, an androgen, or an estrogen can be used.

Table 8-7:   Systemic Chemotherapy: Commonly Reported Reactions

Cutaneous
- Hyperpigmentation of skin (5-fluouraracil, methotrexate)
- Alopecia
- Hand foot syndrome–palmar-plantar erythrodysthesia seen routinely with capecitabine
- Rash—associated with paclitaxel
- Pruritis—of palms/plantar regions described especially with paclitaxel
- Desquamation—described with taxanes

Neurologic
- Ataxia—well described but uncommon with 5-fluorouracil
- Paresthesias—with taxanes (paclitaxel and docetaxel) and described with carboplatin
- Impaired cognitive function—described especially with adjuvant therapy that manifests as difficulty with concentration and recent memory loss
- Pain—described with paclitaxel in joints and long bones
  - At sites of known metastases with vinorelbine use

Gastrointestinal
- Mucositis
- Nausea/emesis less problematic with antiemetics
  - Ondansetron (Zofran®)
  - Granisetron (Kytril®)
  - Aprepitant (Emend®)
- Diarrhea common with capecitabine

Ocular
- Eye tearing—associated with 5-fluorouracil and taxanes
  - Felt to be secondary to stenosis of the lacrimal duct
- Conjunctivitis (5-fluorouracil)

Table 8-7: continued

Cardiac
- Arrhythmia and cardiomyopathy—anthracyclines
- Cardiomyopathy—trastuzumab
- Anthracycline plus taxanes plus trastuzumab (currently under investigation)
- Dexrazoxane with anthracyclines confers protection
- Pegylated liposomal doxorubicin is less cardiotoxic than doxorubicin
- Anthracycline plus taxanes are associated with a decline in LVEF during treatment that recovers over time

Hypersensitivity reactions
- Described with paclitaxel-polyoxylated 35 caster oil solvent base; premedication with steroids reduces risk

New agents currently under investigation are designed to have fewer toxicities and high therapeutic indices

LVEF, left ventricular ejection fraction.

- If a patient has prior exposure to endocrine therapy, first-line tamoxifen followed by fulvestrant, or tamoxifen followed by an aromatase inhibitor is a suggested sequence.
- In the case of prior exposure to fulvestrant, the sequential pathway may include a nonsteroidal fol-

Table 8-8: Endocrine Therapy Approach to Metastatic Breast Cancer

Premenopausal	Postmenopausal
Tamoxifen	Tamoxifen
Fulvestrant	Fulvestrant
	Aromatase inhibitors
	(steroidal exemestane, nonsteroidal letrozole, and anastrozole)
	Megestrol
	Androgens
	Estrogens

lowed by a steroidal aromatase inhibitor followed by megestrol followed by an androgen or an estrogen.

- Patients with brief response to prior hormonal therapy or those with visceral crises at presentation, in general, should be given an initial trial of chemotherapy.

▪ Special Conditions in MBC

- Bone metastases
  - Frequent complications are an indication of systemic spread.
  - Occur in up to 70% of patients having advanced breast or prostate cancer
  - Both osteolytic and osteoblastic lesions can occur.
  - Most breast tumors are predominantly osteolytic; 15–20% are predominantly osteoblastic.
  - Secondary formation of bone occurs in response to bone destruction (hence a positive bone scan can be seen in osteolytic disease).
  - Tumor cells in breast cancer exhibit osteoclast-inducing characteristics, which leads to bone resorption and the release of growth factors from the bone matrix.
  - On average, 20% of patients are alive 5 years after a diagnosis of bone metastases.
  - Consequences of bone metastases include:
    - Pain, immobility, and functional impairment
    - Pathologic fractures (osteolytic and osteoblastic) associated with increased mortality
    - Hypercalcemia associated with:
      - Lethargy
      - Nausea
      - Vomiting
      - Renal insufficiency/failure
    - Nerve compression syndromes
      - Spinal cord compression
      - Bowel/bladder dysfunction
    - Need for surgery with or without radiation for palliation and treatment of bone lesions, pathologic fractures, and cord compression

- Biochemical markers as a measure of bone turnover and a means for following patients with MBC under investigation are:
  - Osteoblastic lesions (tumors secrete osteoblastic-activating factor, which leads to new bone deposition in areas where there has not been prior resorption)
    - Bone-specific alkaline phophatase
    - Osteocalcin
    - C-propeptide type 1 procollagen
  - Osteolytic lesions (tumors secrete factors that stimulate osteoclastic maturation and activity, leading to increased resorption of bone. The resorption of bone in turn releases growth factors that stimulate additional osteoclastic activity)
    - C-terminal telopeptide of type 1 collagen*
    - Tartrate-resistant acid phophatase
    - Urinary N-telopeptide levels*

(*Most useful so far.)
  - Role of bisphosphonates
    - Bisphosphonates play an important role in the breast cancer patient, with several areas of use:
      - Skeletal metastases and imaging evidence of bone destruction
      - Maintenance of normal bone health, as more patients are surviving and as therapies induce menopause
      - Adjuvant setting
    - Bind to bone mineral and prevent tumor from adhering to bone (interfere with adhesion to bone matrix)
    - Prevent osteoclastic-mediated bone resorption by restricting bone-derived growth factors, and interfere with maturation of osteoclasts
    - Inhibit matrix metalloproteinases
    - Interrupts the sclerotic activity of osteoblasts
    - Have an antiproliferative effect on tumor cells
    - Able to reduce bone events when used at the time of diagnosis of skeletal metastases
    - Most data derived from studies of IV bisphosphonates pamidronate and zoledronic acid

- Both are US Food and Drug Administration (FDA)-approved for:
  - Hypercalcemia of malignancy
  - Bone metastases from breast cancer
- Infusion times differ
  - Zoledronic acid—15 minutes
  - Pamidronate—2 hours
- Zoledronic acid dose must be reduced when there is evidence of renal insufficiency. Pamidronate dose should also be reduced.
- An oral bisphosphonate preparation (clodronate) is available in Europe and Canada.
- Both forms reduce skeletal events in patients already documented to have osteolytic lesions. NSAB B-34 trial is testing clodronate vs. placebo in the adjuvant setting to, hopefully, confirm earlier studies demonstrating a prevention effect.
- Also under investigation are antibodies to parathyroid hormone-related protein (PTHrP) and osteopro-tegerin.
- Adjuvant therapy for breast cancer and the role of bisphosphonates
  - Treatment of breast cancer in the adjuvant setting involves
    - Chemotherapy
    - Endocrine therapy
      - SERMS
      - Aromatase inhibitors
      - Ovarian ablation
        - Surgery
        - Chemical (LHRH agonists)
    - All have a central effect of estrogen depletion, which leads to a decline in bone mineral density due to bone loss and decreased quality of bone.
    - Treatment-induced menopause ranges from 40–71% with either anthracycline- or methotrexate-based regimens.
- Brain metastases/carcinomatosis meningitis
  - More commonly seen in HER-2/neu-overexpressing tumors treated with trastuzumab that are responding peripherally

- Consultations with appropriate teams should be obtained:
  - Neurology
  - Neurosurgery
  - Radiation oncology
- Therapy is usually a multimodality approach and may include:
  - Whole brain radiation
  - Stereotatic radiation
  - Resection of isolated lesions
  - Debulking of disease in select cases
  - Intrathecal therapy through a ventricular reservoir
- If carcinomatosis meningitis is suspected, it is necessary to obtain documentation with a cerebral spinal fluid (CSF) examination.
  - Up to three lumbar punctures may be necessary to optimize attempts at a diagnosis.
- Occasionally characteristic radiograph changes suggesting leptomeningeal involvement, will appear on MRI. In this setting, suspicious CSF cytology results may be adequate for diagnosis and treatment.
- Treatment can include intrathecal methotrexate 12 mg weekly until maximal clinical response is achieved, then biweekly administration.
- Other useful intrathecal drugs include thiotepa and cytosine arabinoside (ara-C).

- Spinal cord compression
  - 5% of patients with breast cancer develop cord compression.
  - Treatment involves dexamethasone 100 mg IV bolus followed by tapering to a maintenance dose.
  - Trimethoprim/sulfamethoxazole (TMX/SMX) prophylaxis for *Pneumocystic carinii* pneumonia is also important.
  - Radiotherapy administration is considered the mainstay of treatment.
  - Rare indications for neurosurgery include:
    - Denovo presentation
    - Progression of disease in the face of prior radiation

■ References

1.   Slamon DJ, Leyland-Jones B, Shak S, et al. Use of chemotherapy plus a monoclonal antibody against HER2 for metastatic breast cancer that overexpresses HER2. *N Engl J Med.* 2001;344:783-792.

2.   Marty M et al. Randomized phase II trial of the efficacy and safety of trastuzumab combined with docetaxel in patients with human epidermal growth factor receptor-2-positive metastatic breast cancer administered as first line treatment: the M77001 study group. *JCO* 2005;23:4265-4274.

3.   Extra J, Cognetti F, Maraninchi R, et al. Long-term survival demonstrated with trastuzumab plus docetaxel: 24 month data from a randomised trial (M77001) in HER2-positive metastatic breast cancer. *J Clin Oncol.* 2005;23(suppl):17s.

4.   Roodman GD. Mechanisms of bone metastasis. *N Engl J Med.* 2004;350:1655-1664.

CHAPTER 9

Long-Term Complications

■ Cardiac Risks (Table 9-1)

- Factors contributing to therapy-related cardiac dysfunction in the breast cancer patient
  - Chemotherapy agents (anthracyclines, taxanes)
  - Targeted therapy (trastuzumab)[1,2]
  - Patient's age
  - Multimodality therapies (eg, chemotherapy and radiation)
  - Preexisting heart disease

■ Increased Incidence of Second Malignancies

- May occur decades after adjuvant chemotherapy, breast irradiation, and tamoxifen
- Radiation therapy to chest wall
  - Associated with a slight increase in development of lung cancer and sarcomas
  - Malignancies can occur 10 or more years following therapy
- Chemotherapy
  - Alkylating agents (cyclophosphamide) and topoisomerase II inhibitors doxorubicin and epirubicin are associated with:
    - Myeloid leukemias
    - Myelodysplastic syndrome (MDS)
- Postadjuvant therapy incidence up to 2.5%[3]
- Update of the overall EBCTCG meta-analysis[4] finds when comparing anthracycline-based regimens vs. no chemotherapy or methotrexate-based treatments vs. CMF-based chemotherapy is associated with an excess mortality of about 0.2% from leukemia or lymphoma or heart disease during an average 6 years of follow-up.

Table 9-1: **Cardiac Risk with Trastuzumab in Combination with Anthracyclines and Taxanes*[a]**

Drug	Incidence (%)
Trastuzumab	3–7
Trastuzumab plus paclitaxel	13
Trastuzumab plus cyclophosphamide and anthracycline	27
Paclitaxel plus anthracycline[†,b,c]	8
Paclitaxel	1

*Etiology decreased clearance of doxorubicin when given shortly before paclitaxel; not seen with docetaxel.[b]

[†]Limiting maximal dose of doxorubicin to 380 mg/m^2 allows doxorubicin and paclitaxel to be administered safely.[c]

[a]Seidman A, Hudis C, Pierri MK, et al. Cardiac dysfunction in the trastuzumab clinical trials experience. *J Clin Oncol.* 2002;20:1215-1221.

[b]Valero V, Perez E, Dieras V. Doxorubicin and taxane combination regimens for metastatic breast cancer: focus on cardiac effects. *Semin Oncol.* 2001;28(suppl12):15-23.

[c]Loerzel VW, Dow KH. Cardiac toxicity related to cancer treatment. *Clin J Oncol Nurs.* 2003;7:557-562.

■ References

1. Seidman A, Hudis C, Pierri MK, et al. Cardiac dysfunction in the trastuzumab clinical trials experience. *J Clin Oncol.* 2002;20:1215-1221.
2. Theodoulou M, Seidman AD. Cardiac effects of adjuvant therapy for early cancer. *Semin Oncol.* 2003;30:730-739.
3. Bernard-Marty C, Cardoso F, Piccart MJ. Use and abuse of taxanes in the management of metastatic breast cancer. *Eur J Cancer.* 2003;39:1978-1989.
4. Early Breast Cancer Trialists "Collaborative Group. Effects of chemotherapy and hormonal therapy for early breast cancer on recurrence and a 15-year survival: an overview of the randomised trials. *Lancet.* 2005;365:1687-1717.

CHAPTER 10

Future Therapeutic Directions

▪ Targeted Therapy in Breast Cancer

- In recent years, there has been a radical shift in treatment, from nonspecific cytotoxic agents to clinical trials of therapies targeted against molecular mechanisms in the growth and development of cancer cells.
  - Defined as therapy directed against a specific known molecular mechanism—the target
  - The target is unique and important in the development of cancer progression.
- Representative targets in breast cancer
  - HER/erbB tyrosine kinase
  - Small molecule tyrosine kinase
  - Angiogenesis
  - Proteinases
  - Vascular endothelial growth factor (VEGF)
  - erbB receptor-tyrosine kinase (RTK) family includes the following transmembrane glycoproteins:
    - $erbB_1$ (EGFR or HER-1)
    - $erbB_2$ (HER-2)
    - $erbB_3$ (HER-3)
    - $erbB_4$ (HER-4)
  - All have a ligand-binding extracellular region and an intracellular region with the RTK activity.
  - The frequency of EGFR overexpression in breast cancer in unknown.
  - HER-2 and EGFR are frequently coexpressed in breast cancer (10–36%).
    - This coexpression is associated with a less favorable prognosis[1] (rationale for targeting).
  - Monoclonal antibodies (MoAbs) are developed that competitively bind to EGFR and inhibit RTK activity (eg, cetuximab).

- Small molecule tyrosine kinase inhibitors
  - Block EGFR signaling by inhibiting adenosine triphosphate (ATP)-binding site of the tyrosine kinase (RTK)
  - Small molecules specific for the EGFR RTK in clinical trials:
    - ZD1839, gefitinib (Iressa®)
    - OSI-774, elotinib (Tarceva®)
  - Gefitinib (oral preparation)
    - Potent antineoplastic activity in several tumors, including breast[1,2]
    - HER-2/neu-overexpressing cell lines are very sensitive to this agent.
    - Preclinical data demonstrate synergy with trastuzumab.
    - Gefitinib enhances the cytotoxicity of taxanes, platinum-based agents, and topotecan.[1]
    - In spite of the above, preliminary results of a phase II trial were not favorable, possibly because patients participating were all heavily pretreated.[2,3]
  - Erlotinib
    - Oral preparation
    - Reversibly inhibits EGFR tyrosine kinase phosphorylation
    - Most common toxicities are acneiform rash (responds to antibiotics) and diarrhea
  - HER-2 (erbB2)
    - Overexpressed in 25–30% of all breast cancers
    - Overexpression is associated with poor outcome.
    - HER-2 is one of the most important targets studied in breast cancer.
    - Original trial with trastuzumab added to chemotherapy demonstrated a DFS benefit (see Figure 5-8).
    - To date, efficacy is established for patients with HER-2/neu-overexpressing MBC.
    - Synergy exists with a variety of chemotherapy agents (see Table 8-4).
    - Use in the adjuvant setting is currently being investigated in well-designed cooperative group clinical trials (see Figure 5-8).

- Questions still unanswered
  - Optimum duration of therapy
    (Note: There is no scientific basis for continuing
    trastuzumab following disease progression.)
  - Optimum dose schedule
    - Weekly and every-3-week schedules are now
      equally efficacious.
  - Optimum method to detect HER-2/neu overex-
    pression
    - Current method is IHC 3+ polyclonal antibody
      staining (Hercep® test, DakoCytomation Inc,
      Carpinteria, CA) (range 0–3+).
      - A score of less than 3+ is confirmed with
        FISH testing (positive result is a ratio of 2.0
        or greater).
- Angiogenesis
  - New capillary formation from existing blood vessels
    plays an important role in the growth of cancer.
  - Theoretically, targeting angiogenesis could be of clini-
    cal value.
- Proteinases
  - Matrix metalloproteinases (MMPs) facilitate the
    destruction of basement membrane and surrounding
    tissue.
  - In the experimental model, inhibition of MMP activ-
    ity can lead to decreased angiogenesis and lowered
    metastatic potential.
  - An optimum model to test MMP inhibition may be
    following chemotherapy or surgery.
  - To date, results of such studies have been disap-
    pointing.
  - Marimastat, the MMP inhibitor tested in breast can-
    cer, produced significant musculoskeletal toxicities.
- VEGF
  - Serum VEGF levels are overexpressed in primary and
    MBC tumors.
  - Higher levels are associated with:
    - Chemotherapy resistance
    - More aggressive natural history
    - Poor prognosis in early-stage breast cancer

- VEGF and signaling pathways that have been targeted by trials of investigational agents include:
  - VEGF glycoprotein (bevacizumab)
    - Humanized MoAb directed against VEGF
    - 9% response rate as monotherapy for refractory MBC
    - Studied as a single agent and in combination with chemotherapy (capecitabine as well as paclitaxel)
    - Capecitabine plus bevacizumab is:
      - Not associated with significant bleeding
      - Well tolerated
      - Most commonly associated with hypertension and proteinuria
    - Objective response or clinical benefit in 17% of patients with advanced cancer at 22 weeks[4]
    - In breast cancer, paclitaxel with or without bevacizumab has been studied as first-line therapy for locally recurrent or metastatic disease.[5] Findings included:
      - 715 eligible patients
      - Response rate of 28.2% for patients receiving paclitaxel–bevacizumab combination vs. paclitaxel alone
      - PFS (progression free survival) of 10.97 months for paclitaxel–bevacizumab combination and 6.11 months for paclitaxel alone
      - HR for the OS was 0.674 in favor of paclitaxel–bevacizumab.
    - Toxicities included:
      - 13% grade 1 hypertension with bevacizumab–paclitaxel and none with paclitaxel alone
      - 2.4% grade 3–4 proteinuria with bevacizumab–paclitaxel and none with paclitaxel alone
    - This trial concluded that the addition of bevacizumab to paclitaxel:
      - Prolongs progression free survival
      - Increases the objective response rate
  - Longer follow-up is needed to assess the OS impact.

- Endothelial cell receptors for VEGF
- Postreceptor protein products
- Endothelial toxins
  - A class of compounds that can selectively inhibit cell migration is currently under investigation.
  - Agents that can disrupt the tumor's endothelial cytoskeleton are also under development.

■ References

1. Ciardiello F, Caputo R, Bianco R, et al. Antitumor effect and potentiation of cytotoxic drugs activity in human cancer cells by ZD-1839 (Iressa), an epidermal growth factor receptor-selective tyrosine kinase inhibitor. *Clin Cancer Res* 2000;6:2053-2063.

2. Schneider BP, Houck WA, Sledge G. Targeted therapy in breast cancer. In: Kaklamani VG, Gradishar WJ, eds. *Diseases of the Breast Updates.* 2nd ed. 2003;6:1-16.

3. Robertson JFR, Gutteridge E, Cheung K, et al. Gefitinib is active in acquired tamoxifen-resistent oestrogen receptor-positive and ER negative breast cancer: results from a phase II study [abstract]. *Proc Am Soc Clin Oncol.* 2003;22:7. Abstract 24.

4. Gordon MS, Margolin K, Talpaz M, et al. Phase I safety and pharmacokinetic study of recombinant human anti-vascular endothelial growth factor in patients with advanced cancer. *J Clin Oncol.* 2001;19:843-850.

5. Miller KD, Wang M, Gralow J, et al. E2100: a randomized phase III trial of paclitaxel versus paclitaxel plus bevacizumab as first-line therapy for locally recurrent or metastatic breast cancer [abstract]. Abstract presented at: Annual Meeting of American Society of Clinical Oncology; May 15, 2005; Orlando, FL.

CHAPTER 11

Special Conditions: Male Breast Cancer, Pregnancy-Associated Cancer, and Cancer in the Elderly

■ Carcinoma of the Male Breast[1,2]

- Accounts for less than 1% of all breast cancer
- Mean age at diagnosis is 58–62 years
- Usually diagnosed by physical exam
- Men do not routinely have mammograms.
- Pathology
  - Similar to breast cancer in women
  - Most common histology is infiltrating ductal carcinoma
  - No statistical difference in comparison with female breast cancer with respect to multicentric disease or the presence of lymphatic invasion
  - More likely to be an estrogen receptor-poor tumor
- Survival does not differ significantly based on gender
- Systemic treatment options mirror female treatment (chemotherapy/endocrine manipulation).
- Surgical standard of care is modified radical mastectomy.
- Clinical genetics consultation should be considered in families with male relatives having breast cancer.

■ Pregnancy-Associated Breast Cancer

- Breast cancer diagnosis during pregnancy
  - Often difficult to diagnose
  - Frequently presents as mastitis in the setting of breast-feeding
  - Most present as painless mass noted by the patient

- Physical examination is often difficult because the breast may be:
  - Engorged
  - Nodular
  - Hypervascular
- Mammography is often not helpful, due to:
  - Glandular nature of the tissue
  - Lactation
- Ultrasound may be a better screening test
- Histologic confirmation still necessary for a definite diagnosis
- Important to take an active approach and essential to make a histologic diagnosis
- General approach, when possible, is to treat the cancer and allow the pregnancy to proceed
- Treatment is often individualized, with the therapeutic approach being the result of weighing the risk to the fetus against the benefits to the mother.

- Pregnancy following diagnosis of breast cancer
  - No prospective studies evaluating the effects of pregnancy after a breast cancer diagnosis
  - Results of studies involving patients with a history of breast cancer are controversial.[3–5]
    - Pregnancy within 2 years of treatment had an adverse effect on breast cancer risk.
    - This was not confirmed in several retrospective studies.

- Effect of adjuvant breast cancer therapy on subsequent fertility
  - Cyclophosphamide leads to amenorrhea through direct ovarian suppression.
  - 5-Fluorouracil and methotrexate are less associated with ovarian failure.
  - Little data exist regarding doxorubicin.
  - The younger a patient is at the time of treatment, the greater the number of oocytes available post-chemotherapy.
  - The return of menses and ovulation is a function of:
    - Age
    - Therapy dose
    - Duration of treatment

- CMF regimen has more of an ovarian suppression effect than AC; the mechanism is related to the duration of therapy.
- Patients on tamoxifen can become pregnant.
- The effect on human fetal development is unknown.
- Women wishing to become pregnant should stop tamoxifen use several months to 1 year before conception.
- In the absence of a recurrence, women who become pregnant after breast cancer treatment should be managed as other pregnant women.

Cancer in the Elderly

- The fastest growing group in the US population is composed of persons older than 65 years of age.
- Cancer is the leading cause of death in the 60–79-year-old group.
- With the increasing cancer incidence in the elderly subset coupled with the increase in life span, cancer in the elderly has become more common.
- Select octogenarians can benefit from surgery and adjuvant treatment.[6]
- Several studies demonstrate that chemotherapy toxicities are not greater in persons older than 65 years of age, indicating that age alone is not a contraindication to chemotherapy.[7–9] The older-than-65-year-old age group can do as well as younger patients, provided supportive care is available.
- Older patients should be assessed initially to identify:
  - Those likely to die of cancer
  - Those with a short life expectancy
- Issues related to the management of the elderly with cancer include:
  - Geriatric assessment
  - Prevention or minimization of toxicities of therapy
  - Management of disease-specific issues
- The National Comprehensive Cancer Network (NCCN) has established a guideline for assessing these issues (NCCN Practice Guidelines in Oncology—v.1.2005).[10]
- It is most important to assess the risk–benefit ratio.

- Consider whether the:
  - Patient is able to tolerate cancer treatment
  - Patient is at risk for complications related to cancer during his or her lifetime
  - Patient will die from the cancer
- The appropriate elderly patient must be selected for treatment administration.
- Anticipated benefits include:
  - Prolonged survival
  - Maintenance of quality of life
  - Palliation of symptoms
- Risks associated with cancer treatment in the elderly
  - Treatment complications (eg, surgery, chemotherapy, radiation)
  - It is important to assure that adequate support is available during chemotherapy administration because of the potential for complications.
    - Neutropenic fever
    - Anemia
    - Mucositis
    - Neurotoxicity
    - Cardiac toxicity
    - Older patients are at risk for severe/prolonged myelosuppression and mucositis; hematopoietic growth factors are effective in patients older than 70 years of age.
  - Other factors to consider:
    - Cognitive functioning
    - Balance
    - Hearing
    - Visceral condition
    - Emotional stability
  - Life expectancy can be assessed by using life-table data.[11]
  - The best guide for judging whether or not cancer treatment is appropriate is to carefully assess the patient using guidelines such as those listed in the 2004 NCCN Senior Adult Oncology Clinical Practice Guidelines.

■ References

1.   Heller KS, Rosen PP, Schottenfeld D, Ashikari R, Kinne DW. Male breast cancer: a clinicopathologic study of 97 cases. *Ann Surg.* 1978;188:60-65.

2.   Borgen PI, Senie RT, McKinnon WM, Rosen PP. Carcinoma of the male breast: analysis of prognosis compared with matched female patients. *Ann Surg Oncol.* 1977;4:385-388.

3.   Von Schoultz E, Johansson H, Wilking N, Rutavist LE. Influence of prior and subsequent pregnancy on breast cancer prognosis. *J Clin Oncol.* 1995;13:430-434.

4.   Sankila R, Heinavaara S, Hakulinen T. Survival of breast cancer patients after subsequent term pregnancy: "healthy mother effect." *Am J Obstet Gynecol.* 1994;170:818-823.

5.   Sutton R, Buzdar AU, Hortobagyi GN. Pregnancy and offspring after adjuvant chemotherapy in breast cancer patients. *Cancer.* 1990;65:847-850.

6.   Extermann M. Management issues for elderly patients with breast cancer. *Curr Treat Options Oncol.* 2004;5:161-169.

7.   Christman K, Muss HB, Case LD, Stanley V. Chemotherapy of metastatic breast cancer in the elderly. The Piedmont Oncology Association experience [see comment]. *JAMA.* 1992;268:57-62.

8.   Sargent DJ, Goldberg RM, Jacobson SD, et al. A pooled analysis of adjuvant chemotherapy for resected colon cancer in elderly patients. *N Engl J Med.* 2001;345:1091-1097.

9.   Chen H, Cantor A, Meyer J, et al. Can older cancer patients tolerate chemotherapy? A prospective pilot study. *Cancer.* 2003;97:1107-1114.

10.   National Comprehensive Cancer Network. Senior Adult Oncology Guidelines v.1.2005. Available at www.nccn.org/professionals/physician_gls/PDF/senior.pdf. Accessed 6/1/05.

11.   Walter LC, Covinsky KE. Cancer screening in elderly patients: a framework for individualized decision making. *JAMA.* 2001;285:2750-2756.

CHAPTER 12

Prevention Trials

■ Breast Cancer Prevention

- EBCTCG
  - Worldwide overview analysis of 55 randomized trials
  - 37,000 women in two-arm randomized study of tamoxifen vs. no treatment
    - Reported breast cancer risk reduction benefit for tamoxifen in hormone receptor-positive tumors because the study was a randomization of tamoxifen vs. no treatment and patients with hormone receptor-positive tumors benefit from tamoxifen.
- NSABP-P1 reported the results of 13,338 premenopausal and postmenopausal women at high risk for breast cancer[1] randomized to tamoxifen or placebo.
  - At 49 months, a benefit was demonstrated for tamoxifen regardless of menopausal status.
  - A benefit was also documented in patients having atypical ductal hyperplasia and LCIS.
  - An added benefit in bone fracture risk reduction was also reported.
- Current prevention trial (NSABP-P2) involves randomization to raloxifene or tamoxifen. Eligibility is based on age, risk assessment, and histologic markers of risk.

■ Reference

1. Fisher B, Costantino JP, Wickerham DL, et al. Tamoxifen for prevention of breast cancer: report of the National Surgical Adjuvant Breast and Bowel Project P-1 Study. *J Natl Cancer Inst.* 1998;90:1371-1388.

CHAPTER 13

Hereditary Breast Cancer

■ Clincal Genetics

- Hereditary breast–ovarian cancer
  - Only a small portion of all breast and ovarian cancer diagnoses are secondary in hereditary predispositions.
  - Sporadic cancers account for the majority of breast cancer cases (85%).
  - Typical history of familial breast cancer may include:
    - Two or more first- or second-degree relatives affected by the same type of cancer
    - An age of onset not usually earlier than expected
  - Familial cancer accounts for 10% of diagnosed cases.
- Hereditary breast cancer
  - Accounts for 5–10% of all cases of breast cancer
  - Hereditary ovarian cancer accounts for 10% of all ovarian cancer.
  - Hereditary breast and ovarian cancers are associated with mutations in BRCA1 and BRCA2 genes.
    - Inherited mutations in BRCA1 and BRCA2 can occur in all races and ethnic groups.
    - Certain populations are at greater risk for inheriting specific mutations in BRCA1 and BRCA2 genes.
      - Within the Ashkenazi Jewish population, 1 out of 40 people have inherited 1 or 2 mutations.
- Recommended screening for high-risk families with hereditary breast and ovarian cancer
  - Breast cancer surveillance beginning at age 18 years for women at highest risk
  - Annual mammography beginning at age 25 years
  - Clinical breast exams every 3–6 months beginning at age 25 years

- Ovarian cancer screening (pelvic exam, transvaginal color Doppler sonography, CA-125) every 6 months beginning at age 35 years
- Women with familial breast cancer less suggestive of hereditary breast cancer may also benefit from similar screening guidelines.

- Risk-reducing surgery
  - Mastectomy and bilateral salpingo-oophorectomy (BSO) may significantly reduce risk but not eliminate it totally.
    - Following BSO, CA-125 should still be monitored because of the small risk of peritoneal cancer.
  - Women with mutations in BRCA1 and BRCA2 genes are at increased risk for contralateral breast cancer.

- BRCA1 gene
  - Located on chromosome 17q
  - Mutations account for 45% of hereditary breast cancer.
  - Mutations are associated with increased risk of:
    - Breast cancer
    - Ovarian cancer
    - Colon cancer
    - Prostate cancer
  - Women carrying BRCA1 mutations have:
    - 85% lifetime risk of developing breast cancer
    - 40–60% lifetime risk of developing ovarian cancer
  - General population risk
    - 12.5% risk of breast cancer
    - 1–2% risk of ovarian cancer
  - Men with BRCA1 mutations are also at risk for developing breast cancer as well as prostate cancer.
  - Men and women with BRCA1 mutations are at a slight increased risk for developing colon cancer by age 70 years.

- BRCA2 gene
  - Located on chromosome 13q
  - Mutations account for 35% of families with hereditary breast cancer.
  - Breast cancer risk probably less than that with BRCA1 mutation

- Up to a 27% risk of ovarian cancer by age 70 years
- 5–10% lifetime risk of breast cancer for males
- Other cancers associated with BRCA2 mutations
  - Pancreas
  - Melanoma

■ Prostate Screening

■ Recommended for males in families with BRCA1 and BRCA2 mutations
  - Should start at age 40–50 years
  - Screening methodology
    - Digital rectal exam
    - Prostate-specific antigen (PSA)

CHAPTER 14

Primary Care Issues for Breast Cancer Survivors

■ Primary Care Issues

- ■ Survivors of breast cancer have unique health issues.
  - ● Routine follow-up to monitor for breast cancer recurrence
  - ● Toxicity from treatment (eg, bone density issues, early menopause)
  - ● Childbearing decisions and effects
  - ● Psychosocial issues regarding coping with the diagnosis and treatment
- ■ Recommended routine follow-up for breast cancer survivors (Table 14-1)
  - ● Most recurrences are detected within the first 5 years, although late recurrences are not uncommon.[1]
  - ● Most recurrences are detected by abnormalities on physical examination or by symptoms.[2,3]
  - ● Follow-up visits should be more frequent early on and should include:
    - ■ Detailed history
    - ■ Detailed physical examination
  - ● Common sites of recurrence include the chest wall, lymph nodes, and breast.
  - ● Important to remember that in the asymptomatic patient, laboratory and radiographic diagnostics rarely identify metastases
  - ● 15–25% of all cases of metastatic breast cancer are asymptomatic recurrences.[4]
  - ● Outside of an investigational trial, there is no justification for measuring tumor markers at regular intervals in asymptomatic patients.[5]
  - ● The estimated risk of a second primary cancer in the contralateral breast is 0.5–1% per year,[6] with the risk

Table 14-1: American Society of Clinical Oncology Breast Cancer Surveillance Guidelines Summary

Recommended Breast Cancer Surveillance

History/eliciting of symptoms

All women should have a careful history every 3 to 6 months for the first 3 years after primary therapy, then every 6 to 12 months for the next 2 years, and then annually.

Physical examination

All women should have a careful physical examination every 3 to 6 months for the first 3 years, then every 6 to 12 months for the next 2 years, and then annually.

Breast self-examination

It is prudent to recommend that all women perform monthly breast self-examination.

Mammography

It is prudent to recommend that all women with a prior diagnosis of breast cancer have yearly mammographic evaluation. Women treated with breast-conserving therapy should have their first posttreatment mammogram 6 months after completion of radiotherapy, then annually or as indicated for surveillance of abnormalities. If stability of mammographic findings is achieved, mammography can be performed yearly thereafter.

Patient education regarding symptoms of recurrence

Since the majority of recurrences occur between scheduled visits, it is prudent to inform women about symptoms of recurrence.

Coordination of care

The majority of breast cancer recurrences will have occurred within the first 5 years after primary therapy. Subsequent care of the patient following primary treatment should be coordinated and not duplicated. In addition, continuity of care should be encouraged and conducted by a physician experienced in the surveillance of cancer patients and in the examination of women with both irradiated and normal contralateral breasts.

Pelvic examination

It is prudent to recommend that all women have a pelvic examination at regular intervals. Longer intervals may be appropriate for women who have had a total abdominal hysterectomy and oophorectomy.

Table 14-1:   continued

Breast Cancer Surveillance Testing—Not Recommended

Complete blood cell count
  The data are insufficient to suggest the routine use of complete blood cell counts.

Automated chemistry studies
  The data are insufficient to suggest the routine use of automated chemistry studies.
  Automated chemistry studies include liver and renal function tests and protein, albumin, and calcium level studies.

Chest roentgenography
  The data are insufficient to suggest the routine use of chest radiographs.

Bone scan
  The data are insufficient to suggest the routine use of bone scans.

Ultrasound of the liver
  The data are insufficient to suggest the routine use of liver ultrasounds.

Computed tomography
  The data are insufficient to suggest the routine use of computed tomography.

Breast cancer tumor marker CA 15-3
  The routine use of the CA15-3 tumor marker for breast cancer surveillance is not recommended.

Breast cancer tumor marker carcinoembryonic antigen (CEA)
  The routine use of the tumor marker CEA for breast cancer surveillance is not recommended.

Reprinted with permission from the American Society of Oncology, Smith TJ et al. *JCO.* 17;1080–1082.

being higher in younger patients and those with genetic variants of breast cancer (BRCA2).

- Radiation therapy may slightly increase the risk of cancer in the contralateral breast.[7]
- Mammography is the current standard of care for detecting asymptomatic or contralateral breast cancer.[8,9]

■ Who should be referred for genetic consultation and testing?

- Patients with a strong family history of breast cancer, including:
  ■ Family members with bilateral disease

- Family members diagnosed at a young age (pre-menopausal)
- Family history or personal history of ovarian or colon cancer
- Family history of male breast cancer
- Family and patient of Ashkenazi Jewish ancestry
- Patients with BRCA1 or BRCA2 mutations and node-negative breast cancer may consider contralateral prophylactic mastectomy to have a positive impact on survival.
- Family members of such patients should be offered a surveillance program as well.

■ Complications of Breast Cancer Treatment and Management

- Breast reconstruction
  - Options
    - Implants
    - Tissue flaps
  - Patients should discuss the options thoroughly with a plastic surgeon. The ultimate decision should be based on anatomy and patient preference.
  - No difference in outcome between immediate or delayed reconstruction
  - An examination of the reconstructed breast, look for
    - Rash-like erythematous skin changes
    - Nodular lesions on the skin or in subcutaneous skin
  - Radiation therapy following reconstruction may impair cosmesis.
    - May be associated with more complications, especially if an implant has been inserted
- Lymphedema
  - Incidence of 10–25%
  - Risk related to:
    - Extent of axillary surgery and radiation treatment
      - Sentinel lymph node procedure is associated with decreased risk

- Obesity
- Local cellulitis
- Treatment guidelines
    - Physical therapy consultation should be obtained early on.
        - Conservative management
        - Elevation of arm
        - Use of compression sleeve/glove
- Ways to prevent lymphedema
    - Avoid venipuncture
    - Avoid infection
    - Avoid cuts/abrasions
    - Avoid intense heat
    - Avoid heavy lifting
- Long-term cardiac effects (see earlier discussion of long-term cardiac risks)
    - Routine screening is not customary
    - If findings suggestive of dysfunction, the following are appropriate:
        - Routine management (EKG, ECHO)
        - β-blockers
        - Angiotensin-converting enzyme (ACE) inhibitors
- Bone marrow disorders
    - No methods for screening are available.
    - Should be considered in differential diagnosis in patients with new-onset cytopenia following treatment for breast cancer
- Gynecologic screening (Table 14-2)
    - Tamoxifen, still the gold standard in adjuvant therapy, is associated with a variety of gynecologic effects. Aromatase inhibitors, now becoming the standard of care, have fewer effects.
    - Gynecologic symptoms associated with tamoxifen (Table 14-3 and Table 14-4)

Table 14-2:   Recommended Gynecologic Screening

- Pelvic exam annually
- Transvaginal ultrasound, if clinically indicated

Table 14-3:   Management of Menopausal Symptoms

Agent	Dose	Type of drug & comments
Vitamin E[a]	800 IU daily	Marginal improvement in clinical outcome compared with placebo
Megestrol acetate[b]	20 mg twice daily or 500 mg intra-muscularly every 2 wk	Progestin, 50-90% of patients report 50% decrease in frequency of hot flushes. Concern about use of hormonal agent in survivors of breast cancer
Flouxetine[c]	20 mg daily	Selective serotonin-reuptake inhibitor; statistically significant reduction in frequency and intensity of hot flushes as compared with placebo
Venlafaxine[d]	75 mg daily	Selective serotonin- and norepinephrine-reuptake inhibitor; statistically significant reduction in frequency and intensity of hot flushes as compared with placebo
Paroxetine[e]	20 mg daily	Selective serotonin-reuptake inhibitor; 67% reduction in number of hot flushes; 75% reduction in intensity score
Clonidine	Oral or patch, 0.1 mg daily	Antihypertensive: 10-20% reduction in symptoms compared with placebo, substantial side effects
Ergotamine- and phenobarbital-based preparations	Various	No benefit after 8 wk compared with placebo
Raloxifene	60 mg daily	Selective estrogen receptor modulator; no difference in incidence of hot flushes compared with placebo

Table 14-3:   continued

Agent	Dose	Type of drug & comments
Soy phyto-estrogens	Daily tablets, each containing 50 mg of soy isoflavones	No improvement in hot flushes compared with placebo

Used with the permission of the Massachusetts Medical Society, Waltham, MA. The original source for this material is the *New England Journal of Medicine,* Vol. 343, p. 1091, 2000, published by Massachusetts Medical Society, Waltham, MA

[a]Barton DL, Loprinzi CL, Quella SK, et al. Prospective evaluation of vitamin E for hot flashes in breast cancer survivors. *J Clin Oncol.* 1998;16:495-500.

[b]Loprinzi CL, Michalak JC, Quella Sk, et al. Megestrol acetate for the prevention of hot flashes. *N Engl J Med.* 1994:331:347-352.

[c]Loprinzi Cl, Quella SK, Sloan JA, et al. Preliminary data from a randomized evaluation of fluoxetine (Prozac) for treating hot flashes in breast cancer survivors [abstract]. *Breast Cancer Res Treat.* 1999;57:34.

[d]Loprinzi CL, Kugler JW, Sloan JA, et al. Venlafaxine in management of hot flashes of breast cancer: a randomized controlled trial. *Lancet.* 2000;356:2059-2063.

[e]Stearns V, Issacs C, Crawford J, et al. A pilot trial assessing the efficacy of paroxetine hydrochloride (Paxil) in controlling hot flashes [abstract]. Breast [abstract]. *Breast Cancer Res Treat.* 1998;50:308.

- Hot flushes (not age restricted). Even if patient has previously undergone menopause naturally (not related to chemotherapy), patient may still experience hot flushes with tamoxifen use.
- Night sweats
- Vaginal discharge

Table 14-4:   Vaginal Symptoms

- Lubricant
- Estrogen rings/Estring
- Vaginal estrogen cream (vaginal estradiol)
- Little systemic absorption with vaginal estradiol

- Vaginal dryness and itching
- Hot flushes/night sweats improve with time.
- Menstrual function may remain normal, become disrupted, and/or revert to normal post tamoxifen therapy.
- Tamoxifen increases the risk of endometrial cancer, unlike aromatase inhibitors.
- Endometrial cancer following 5 years of tamoxifen at an incidence up to 2%.[10,11]
- Endometrial cancer is usually low grade and diagnosed at an early stage.
- Benign effects of tamoxifen on endometrium:
  - Thickening
  - Cysts
- Benign changes can preclude screening for cancer, as screening measures are less specific.
- Recommended gynecologic follow-up for patients on tamoxifen
  - Annual pelvic exam
  - Uterine bleeding or abnormal pelvic exam require a complete evaluation, which often includes an endometrial biopsy.
  - Important to keep in mind that in the majority of patients with uterine bleeding, there is a benign cause.
- Postchemotherapy osteoporosis concerns
  - 8% annual bone loss reported in patients following adjuvant chemotherapy[9] in comparison with 1–2% per annum in postmenopausal women not receiving chemotherapy.
  - Etiology is felt to be related to the sudden onset of menopause as well as the individual effects of chemotherapy drugs.[12,13]
  - As with normal menopause, trabecular bone is more affected than cortical bone.[13]
- Tamoxifen and osteoporosis risk
  - Postmenopausal women on tamoxifen may experience BMD improvement over 2 years.

- Young premenopausal women with tamoxifen may experience varying degrees of BMD loss.[14]
- Aromatase inhibitors were associated with a slow decline in BMD over 2 years.
- According to previously reported data from the ATAC trial, anastrozole was associated with BMD loss at the spine and hip, while tamoxifen was associated with an increase in BMD.[15]
- It is unknown whether BMD stabilizes over time.
- ASCO guidelines for BMD screening in breast cancer patients[16]
  - Routine screening is recommended for:
    - All women older than 65 years of age
    - All women aged 60–64 years with:
      - Family history
      - Body weight greater than 70 kg
      - Prior nontraumatic fracture
      - Other risk factors
    - Postmenopausal women of any age receiving aromatase inhibitors
    - Premenopausal women with therapy-associated premature menopause
  - BMD should be repeated yearly after initial exam
  - All patients should be encouraged to participate in an exercise program involving weight-bearing exercises and to take calcium and vitamin D supplements as outlined later.
  - Reported potential toxicities with bisphosphonates need to be monitored.
    - Osteonecrosis of the jaw
    - Renal insufficiency
    - Screen
- Recommendations for managing osteoporosis risks
  - If menopause is induced, BMD should be checked within 6–12 months.
  - Therapy should be initiated to prevent further loss if BMD is 1–2 standard deviations (SDs) below the mean. Individual circumstances should be assessed when considering the use of a bisphosphonate.

- Patients should maintain adequate calcium/vitamin D intake (1,200–1500 mg/day calcium, 800 international units [IU]/day vitamin D)
- Thromboembolic risks
  - Tamoxifen is associated with a small increased risk of deep venous thrombosis (DVT), pulmonary embolism (PE), and stroke (0.5%); may be higher with concurrent endocrine treatment and chemotherapy.
  - Aromatase inhibitors have less or no risk of thromboembolic events (one half the risk of tamoxifen).
- Psychosocial issues
  - The most difficult time for patients is the first year after diagnosis and therapy.
  - Physicians should inquire about fatigue, anxiety, cognitive disorders, sexual dysfunction, and mood disorders.
  - Risk factors for more significant psychosocial problems
    - Preexisting psychosocial condition
    - Younger age
    - Poor body image in conjunction with menopausal symptoms, lymphedema, and weight gain from treatment
  - Patient participation in support groups should be encouraged.

■ References

1. Saphner T, Tormey D, Gray R. Annual hazard rates of recurrence for breast cancer after primary therapy. *J Clin Oncol.* 1996;14:2738-2746.

2. Winchester DP, Sener SF, Khandekar JD, et al. Symptomatology as an indicator of recurrent or metastatic breast cancer. *Cancer.* 1979;43:956-960.

3. Pandya KJ, McFadden ET, Kalish LA, Tormey DC, Taylor SG 4th, Falkson G. A retrospective study of earliest indicators of recurrence in patients on Eastern Cooperative Oncology Group adjuvant chemotherapy trials for breast cancer. A preliminary report. *Cancer.* 1985;55:202-205.

4. Schapira DV, Urban N. A minimalist policy for breast cancer surveillance. *JAMA.* 1991;265:380-382.

5. Clinical practice guidelines for the use of tumor markers in breast and colorectal cancer. *J Clin Oncol.* 1996;14:2843-2877.

6. Dawson LA, Chow E, Goss PE. Evolving perspectives in contralateral breast cancer. *Eur J Cancer.* 1998;34:2000-2009.

7. Boice JO, Harvey EB, Blettner M, Stovall M, Flannery JT. Cancer in the contralateral breast after radiotherapy for breast cancer. *N Engl J Med.* 1992;326:781-785.

8. Mellink WA, Holland R, Hendriks JH, Peeters PH, Rutgers EJ, van Daal WA. The contribution of routine follow-up mammography to an early detection of asynchronous contralateral breast cancer. *Cancer.* 1991;67:1844-1848.

9. Grosse A, Schreer I, Frischbier HJ, Maass H, Loening T, Bahnsen J. Results of breast conserving therapy for early breast cancer and the role of mammographic follow-up. *Int J Radiat Oncol Biol Phys.* 1997;38:761-767.

10. Fisher B, Costantino JP, Wickerham DL, et al. Tamoxifen for prevention of breast cancer: report of the National Surgical Adjuvant Breast and Bowel Project P-1 Study. *J Natl Cancer Inst.* 1998;90:1371-1388.

11. Fisher B, Costantino JP, Redmond CK, Fisher ER, Wickerham DL, Cronin WM. Endometrial cancer in tamoxifen-treated breast cancer patients: findings from the National Surgical Adjuvant Breast and Bowel Project (NSABP) B-14. *J Natl Cancer Inst.* 1994;86:527-537.

12. Shapiro CL, Manola J, Leboff M. Ovarian failure after adjuvant chemotherapy is associated with rapid bone loss in women with early-stage breast cancer. *J Clin Oncol.* 2001;19:3306-3311.

13. Roodman GD. Mechanisms of bone metastasis. *N Engl J Med.* 2004;350:1655-1664.

14. Burstein HJ, Winer EP. Primary care for survivors of breast cancer. *N Engl J Med.* 2000;343:1086-1094.

15. Howell A, on behalf of the ATAC Trialists Group. Effect of anastrozole on bone mineral density: 2-year results of the Arimidex (Anastrozole), Tamoxifen, Alone or in Combination (ATAC) trial [abstract]. *Breast Cancer Res Treat.* 2003; 82(suppl 1):S27. Abstract 129.

16. Hillner BE, Ingle JN, Chlebowski RT, et al. American Society of Clinical Oncology 2003 update on the role of bisphosphonates and bone health issues in women with breast cancer. *J Clin Oncol.* 2003;21:4042-4057.

Index

Note: Page numbers with *f* indicate figures, *t* indicate tables.